BIOENERGETIC BASICS:

The Art of Dynamic Wellness
with Goiz Biomagnetic Pairs

Janice Bailey

This publication is designed to educate and provide general information regarding the subject matter covered. However, laws and practices often vary from state to state and country to country and are subject to change. Because each situation is different, specific advice should be tailored to the particular circumstances. For this reason, the reader is advised to consult with his or her own health advisor regarding that individual's specific situation.

The author has taken reasonable precautions in the preparation of this book and believe the information presented in the book is accurate at publishing. However, neither the author nor the publisher assume any responsibility for any errors or omissions. The author and publisher specifically disclaim any liability resulting from the use or application of the information contained in this book, and the information is not intended to serve as medical advice related to individual situations.

While this guidebook's subject matter can help produce wellness, it is not intended to replace or supplant licensed professional health care. The author is not a licensed physician and offers this guidebook as an educational and research tool only.

ISBN: 1-4392-0259-1
ISBN-13: 9781439202593
Library of Congress Control Number: 2008906145

Visit www.bioenergeticbasics.com to order additional copies.

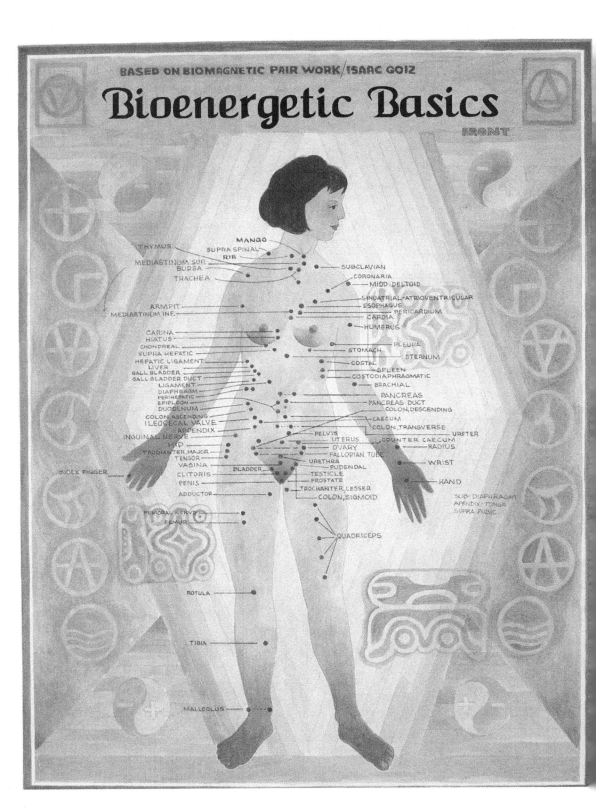

BASED ON BIOMAGNETIC PAIR WORK/ISAAC GOIZ

Bioenergetic Basics

FRONT

Bioenergetic Basics

BASED ON BIOMAGNETIC PAIR WORK OF   ISAAC GOIZ

BACK

NECK
LATISSIMUS DORSI
QUADRATE
LUMBAR
LUMBAR PLEXUS
GLUTEUS
ISCHIUM
ISCHIUM
BRANCH
RENAL CAPSULE

CALYX
ILIAC

FEMUR

POPLITEAL
KNEE LIGAMENT

ACHILLES

DORSAL
SCAPULA
ADRENAL
KIDNEY
CAVA
SACRUM
FLANK
PERIRENAL
PERITONEUM

INTER
ILIAC

COCCYX
RECTUM
ANUS
SCIATIC

CALCANEUS

ILEOCECAL VALVE

CERVICAL

THORACIC

LUMBAR

SACRUM

COCCYX

HEAD
PINEAL
CEREBELLUM

PARIETAL

OCCIPITAL

RACHIDIAN
BULB
ATLAS

CERVICAL
CERVICAL
PLEXUS

Bioenergetic Basics

HEAD

PINEAL

CRANIAL
LACHRYMAL
EYEBROW
EYELID
EYE
CANTHUS
ORBITAL
FLOOR
CHEEKBONE

MAXILAR
NASAL SINUS

NOSE
MAXILLARY
SINUS
MALAR

TONSIL
LARYNX

HYPOTHALAMUS
PITUITARY
SUPRACILIAR
ANTIPOLE
POLE
FOREHEAD
POLYGON
INTERCILIAR
UPPER EAR
EAR
ANGLE

COMMISSURE
TONGUE

◄FRONT

SIDE
▽

THYROID

TEMPORAL

TEMPLE

PARIETAL

CHIASM

MASTOID

BASED ON BIOMAGNETIC
PAIR WORK OF
ISAAC GOIZ

CHIN

MANDIBLE

JUGULAR

PAROTID
VAGUS NERVE
CAROTID
PARATHYROID
STERNOCLEIDO-
MASTOID

From the Book, Bioenergetic Basics written by Janice Bailey

This book is written in partial fulfillment of a challenge Isaac Goiz gave to our class of spring of 2000. After teaching us of his findings, he charged us with informing others, saying that he was not concerned about remuneration, asking only that we give him credit, mentioning his name, much as he did for Dr. Richard Broeringmeyer who preceded him. Hopefully, this book does that, and the author alone takes full responsibility for any errors that might exist.

Dedicated to Craig.

Check out our video on how to scan the body
@ our website:
www.bioenergeticbasics.com

Thank you for your interest in wellness.

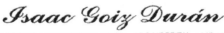

Ced. Prof. 813725   R.F.C. GODI-410413 Q47   OIU-MEX./50-803

To: Professor Janice Bailey, Director   August 9, 2000
    Worldcure
    710 Cypress
    Ranger, Texas 76470

Dear Professor Bailey:

It is with much pleasure that I direct this letter to you. As a student and graduate from the **Centro de Investigacion de Biomagnetismo Medico, S.C.**, and its 5th Curso Nacional de Biomagnetismo Medico, 2000, you have been awarded the highly coveted diploma of graduation which also include the more than 100 hours of practicum in and out of our clinic in Mexico City.

As I indicated, I am happy to give you full authorization to carry forth with your important work with MEDICAL BIOMAGNETISM. This includes your work in bringing forth written materials translated from Spanish to English, such as your excellent rendition of EL PAR BIOMAGNETICO which you carried out. Also, your great efforts in education so as to spread the word to the world about these most efficacious means of reducing suffering which I have spent a lifetime developing.

Not only do we endorse you in your efforts, we offer any help and assistance that you might require in the future in carrying forth the important work you are doing.

Sincerely,

Luis Moya No. 5   Basilio Pérez No. 11 Esq. Juan N. Navarro   Insurgentes Sur No. 107 Séptimo Piso
San Pedro Xalostoc   Col. Constitución de la Rep. C.P. 07469,   Col. Juárez, Zona Rosa
Estado de México   México, D.F. Tel. 5781-8511   México, D.F. C.P. 06600
C.P. 55310 Tel. 5755-8811   Tel.: 52-07-14-52

The above is a copy of a supportive endorsement letter dated August 9, 2000, to Janice Bailey from Isaac Goiz (Duran).

Acknowledgments

Many thanks to Craig Harris and to Leslie Maria Cramer
for innumerable hours of excellent help, editing and suggestions,
to Lucinda Hilbrink for editing on her vacation time,
to Kathy Gordon for her work with the computer, and to Lupita Navarro.

Applause for Fernando Tames and his fine illustrations.

Muchisimas gracias to Isaac Goiz Duran for having persevered in his research of biomagnetic pairs and shared with me.

And a special thank you to all my readers. Helping you to learn how to feel
dynamically well and be more in charge of your health is very gratifying.

Table of Contents

Chapters

INTRODUCTION

Fields of subtle energies inhabit what science has wrongly believed to be the *"vacuum of empty space."* We ourselves are beings of energy and this book is about the **art** of managing that energy for dynamic wellness. Dictionaries say that art is human effort to supplement or alter the work of nature. Physician Isaac Goiz of Mexico City, then, is an artist of energy.

In a class including 28 MDs, 3 nurses, a nun and myself, he demonstrated how working on the unseen subtle energy flow may produce an *oeuvre d'art* equally as moving as a musical masterpiece. One of the students, also an M.D., volunteered to be the canvas upon which Goiz would carry out his art form. The man had been crippled by polio at a young age and wore a prosthesis with a high heel and thick sole on the polio-shortened leg. Goiz placed two magnets on the man and after about 20 minutes, told him, "Get up and walk." His short leg changed length practically before our eyes that day in Mexico City. He no longer needed the prosthesis! Those in the class marveled with the bewildered man who exclaimed with joy, "Doctor, these biomagnetic pairs will change medical history!"

As the Nobel Prize is awarded for discovering how to eradicate a single disease (such as that for stomach ulcers), Goiz could be called and recalled to the stage in Stockholm based on biomagnetic pairs. In 1995 he published *El Par Biomagnetico* (translated as *The Biomagnetic Pair* in 2002 by this author) for which he received recognition from Ecuador's Universidad Nacional de Loja and Mexico's Universidad de Chapingo. Since the first biomagnetic pair discovery in 1988, he has located over 250 pairs for eradicating a plethora of diseases. When *El Par Biomagnetico* was released, there were 114 biomagnetic pairs (BMPs) with 20 special BMPs for a total of 134. In 2002, when the English version was ready, the number of BMPs had increased to over 200. At present there are 267 contained in this guidebook. In the words of Goiz, "these pairs associated with the elements of diagnosis or evaluation permit us to understand and treat practically all human pathologies, including less common syndromes, and tumor phenomena such as cancer." Nevertheless, this method remains basically unknown in the English- speaking world.

The method--the art form--empowers the body to eradicate numerous viral infections for which there are no effective medications. With it the body may easily destroy harmful bacteria such as staphylococcus and streptococcus. It may counter fungus and parasites such as pinworm and clarify troubling health problems we call syndromes. The method also locates and may prevent disease situations from evolving before symptoms arise. The amount of recovery time is shockingly fast, though not necessarily as rapid as with the above-mentioned case of the man with polio.

The absolute ease of this art form is phenomenal. For example, to discover and treat AIDS, adult onset diabetes, benign and cancerous tumors, herpes, and other conditions, he has the person, fully clothed, lie on a table. He places magnets on the corresponding biomagnetic pair locations as specified by his research. Painful exploratory surgery and time-consuming lab tests are rendered unnecessary. Anesthesia and many drugs are not a requirement. Such wellness, then, is truly an art form encouraged through this information and at minimal cost to the patient.

Much like Vivaldi's brilliant violin concertos engage musicians and delight listeners, this art form can transform you. It can give you peace through confidence in being able to participate in more of what is happening within you. Read this entire book as presented before ever attempting depolarizations. In that way you may best learn about and perhaps become an energy artist who creates wellness for yourself, family and friends such that you may never have dreamed!

Disclaimer:

While this guidebook's artform can allow the body to produce wellness, it is not intended to replace or supplant licensed professional health care. The author is not a licensed physician and offers this guidebook as an educational and research tool only.

BIOENERGETIC BASICS:

THE ART OF DYNAMIC WELLNESS
with GOIZ BIOMAGNETIC PAIRS

CHAPTER 1
BACKGROUND OF BIOENERGETIC BASICS

In 1988, the now controversial physician Isaac Goiz (Duran) attended a life-changing session on bioenergy at the medical school of the University of Guadalajara in Mexico. Goiz tells how Dr. Richard Broeringmeyer (see photo, following page) described his work with NASA (National Aeronautic and Space Administration). Broeringmeyer, who passed away in 1991, measured and tested the early astronauts before and after their space mission. He noticed that when the astronauts returned from space, their bodies were slightly lopsided with one leg shortened. (Before going into outer orbit they had been normal.)

Broeringmeyer had speculated about what caused the abnormality. He wondered if it had anything to do with the fact that the astronauts were far from the direct magnetic influence of planet earth. To his delight he found the answer. By applying magnets to their bodies, it caused them to lose the lopsidedness and they regained their normal stance and leg length.*

According to Goiz, Broeringmeyer had continued his studies with magnetism and looked at how it related to pH (acidity and alkalinity) in the body. He developed certain practices based on biomagnetism, which he shared in Guadalajara.

He taught Goiz about biomagnetic energy in the human body and reviewed what he had learned about interference of energy flow.

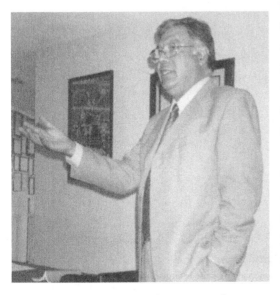

1. Isaac Goiz Duran, Discoverer of Biomagnetic Pairs

Broeringmeyer stressed that organs and tissues in the body can become magnetically polarized. He lectured about his polar therapy based on pH and also about the importance of hydrogen ions in health and disease.

Broeringmeyer's technique involved kinesiology (muscle testing) to locate magnetic polarizations. When he found a polarization, indicated by changes in muscle strength, he would apply a magnet to the indicated area. He suggested leaving the magnet in place for 30 days, as he had done with the astronauts, to obtain depolarization.

As one of the physicians attending the seminar, Goiz was fascinated. Born in 1941, he had lived his whole life in Mexico, at first studying chemical engineering. Later he changed his field, going into medicine as a physical therapist. He incorporated a variety of approaches and studies such as massage and acupuncture in his work. Eventually he studied and became a licensed medical doctor. With his broad background, he was aware that there were many factors about health that were being ignored in the conventional medical school courses. New scientific health findings intrigued him, wherever they came from. He continually sought a wider understanding of the body to improve his expertise in his own medical practice.

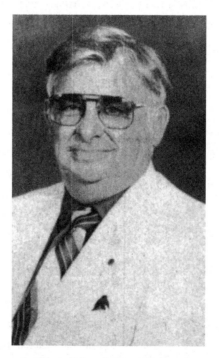

2. Dr. Richard Broeringmeyer

*In the 1930's, Dr. Albert R. Davis discovered the phenomenon of apparent leg length changes and placement of magnets on various body parts. A patent was applied for on December 20, 1976, for his method of conducting a screening and diagnostic examination to identify "damaged, diseased, abnormal and/or malfunctioning parts of the body". Davis's discovery was not mentioned by Goiz in his writings.

CHAPTER 2
AIDS AS CATALYST IN
BIOMAGNETIC PAIR DISCOVERY

Within a week following the Broeringmeyer seminar, Goiz's discovery of the first bio-magnetic pair occurred. He returned to his Mexico City clinic pondering the concepts of Dr. Broeringmeyer. A patient stricken with an advanced case of AIDS soon arrived at his clinic. In 1988 not much was known about the treatment of that devastating disease. Goiz scanned the patient with a magnet by moving it over the body. When he passed the magnet over the thymus area, one side of the body immediately shortened, similar to the lopsided-ness Broeringmeyer had observed in the astronauts.

At that instant something nudged Goiz's intuition. It was an idea beyond what Bro-eringmeyer taught about diseased organs being polarized. Goiz thought that in the case of AIDS there might exist more than just a single polarized area of the body.

Magnetic poles come in pairs, he thought to himself. They are not just a north pole alone or an unaccompanied south pole (which is one limitation of other biomagnetic thera-pies presently being practiced). Perhaps, he postulated, AIDS could be caused by a **PAIR of magnetic poles** or a pair of polarized body areas. If so, the thymus gland below the collar bone could represent one of the poles, since placing a magnet in that location caused a drawing up of one side of the body. The other pole, he reasoned, had to be hidden some-where else. Where, he asked himself, could that other pole be? And, if he were to locate the other pole and put a magnet on it, would the patient's body lose the shortness and return to normal? Would this progressed case of AIDS be affected?

Leaving the first magnet over the thymus, he set to work scanning the rest of the patient's entire body, front and back, with another magnet. With each placement of the second magnet, he checked to determine if the contracted side of the body had returned to normal.

He checked points over the front of the patient's body. No reaction. He checked the arms, legs, and head. Then he began scanning his back side. Finally, when he placed the second magnet over the area at the end of the coccyx, he saw what he was looking for. <u>The man's shortened leg returned to normal.</u> He conjectured the base of the spine might be the point of the second biomagnetic pole for AIDS.

He left each magnet in place on the patient's body for less than an hour, explaining to the man how the technique might possibly help him. However, he did not know for sure what the effect might be. He assured him also that natural magnets such as the ones he was using would not be harmful. He told him to return in one week to be rechecked.

In the words of Goiz *(from Goiz's seminar, spring of 2000)*,
"When the patient came back, he had no symptoms of his disease. He has continued AIDS-free to this time."

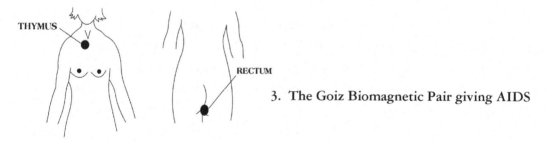

THYMUS

RECTUM

3. The Goiz Biomagnetic Pair giving AIDS

That monumental breakthrough could prove to be one of our most important medical discoveries. The extraordinary concept of the biomagnetic pair, that a sickness has two magnetic poles or points of opposite polarity, was first postulated in 1988:

From Goiz again (The Biomagnetic Pair, p. 15):

"Orthodox medicine of our time conceives pathological phenomena only as unipolar and isolated. But the discovery and practical demonstration of MEDICAL BIO-MAGNETISM . . . confirm(s) physical, biological, and energetic duality of living organisms and . . . their manifestations in health as well as in sickness. That is to say, the pathological and pathogenic manifestations are formed from well-defined poles--positive and negative--or south and north respectively, which depart from the natural limits of organic entropy where health is established as a natural law. That means a constant and biomagnetic resonance exists within the boundaries of health, as well as in the deviations wherein sicknesses originate. So, the presence of one conditions that of the other."

Goiz's dual polarity discovery was the first known example of bioenergetically aiding the body to obliterate an illness with a pair of magnets. That first biomagnetic pair received the name of *Timo/Recto*, (Thymus/Rectum in English.) Goiz said that perhaps the only positive thing about AIDS was that its presence led to the discovery of the main principles of bioenergetic basics: depolarizing biomagnetic pairs with a pair of magnets. There were to be many more firsts. Since that occasion in his Mexico City clinic, Goiz discovered a multitude of applications of depolarizing dual polarities.

"Once I discovered the first pair, I felt that more diseases might respond in the same way. The results were always spectacular."

(Goiz, Mexico City seminar, 2000)

Since the first breakthrough with AIDS, Goiz's research into other biomagnetic pairs in the body has continued. He has helped over 200,000 patients in Mexico, Italy, Ecuador, Peru, Chile and Spain with his art or biomagnetic pair "medicine." Students of Goiz are successfully applying the same principles by utilizing the biomagnetic pairs (BMPs). They depolarize the BMPs as a new, alternative medical treatment in their respective fields of gynecology, dentistry, pediatrics, ophthalmology, psychiatry, etc., often with remarkable positive health benefits.

<u>With the understanding of how disease states exist due to Goiz's newly defined biomagnetic pairs, we take the first step in BIOENERGETIC BASICS.</u> There are no overdoses in this method. It is not expensive. It is not toxic. It does not require lab tests or surgery. The magnetic energy applied cannot harmfully alter the milieu within or around the cell as drugs can. Instead, maintains Goiz, it organizes and stabilizes cells so the body can heal itself.

Benefits of the method are usually seen within one week or sooner depending on the case. Not all conditions respond the same or as quickly as others. But often the patients recover in an unexpectedly short time. Viruses can be eradicated quickly. Bacteria, parasites, and fungi may take longer, but once they are located and identified they are substantially weakened. Then the body's own immune system can destroy them, often without the need for antibiotics or other medications. It has also been found that young children's bodies (and animals') often heal themselves more rapidly with magnets than do adults.

This knowledge about AIDS as well as other "incurable" diseases that has been developed by Goiz needs to be better understood by everyone possessing a body. Bioenergetic basics can help us feel better and learn to be more in control of our bodies. Goiz's work can give us greater understanding about ourselves. Discussing his findings with one's health care providers is a good beginning. Implementing them can reduce fear and dependency and give us confidence and peace.

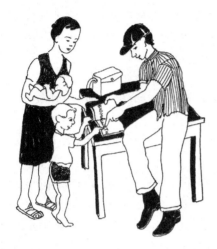

4. Learning about the human body
(from DONDE NO HAY DOCTOR by David Werner, p. 19)

CHAPTER 3
SPEAKER MAGNETS AND LEUKEMIA

The author, who is not a doctor, wanted to help her father who had developed leukemia. Upon learning about the possible benefits from what Goiz was doing, she petitioned him to admit her as his student in early 2000. After studying with him and working under his tutelage at his clinic in Mexico City, she was ready to see what could be done for her father.

Normal white blood cell count is measured from around 4,500 to 10,000 white blood cells (WBC) per microliter, and his count had climbed close to 100,000, at 98,000. Following the bioenergetic basics procedure, she scanned his body. She placed two magnets pulled from second-hand store speakers on the leukemia points, leaving them in place for some 30 minutes.

Her father, a skeptical Ph.D. from an Ivy League university, verified that at his next regularly scheduled blood test his white cell count was down by almost 10,000, which, he considered, might be due merely to remission. But the count continued downward more

Years	95	97	99	2000	2001	2002	2005
White Blood Cells in Thousands							
90				98			
80			80				
70							
60		65					
50					51		
40						41	
30	33						36

than 60,000 over time. (See chart.) It was lowered to 36,000, which seemed to his oncologist quite remarkable for a 92 year old man who had refused conventional treatment. For bioenergetic basics colleagues, remarkableness is often the rule.

If we accept the current findings of science about the nature of matter, it becomes easier to understand how magnets could help the body with leukemia. When we touch our bodies they feel solid to us. They look substantial to our eyes. In spite of what our senses tell us, quantum physics shows us that the body--all matter--is not as solid as we perceive.

Humans are beings composed of atoms held together by the energy of our atoms' electrons. There is a great amount of space between each of our atoms. Additionally, each atom is also mostly space, with (comparatively) vast distances between its center point and its electrons. **We are space and energy.** Much of what is reported in this book about the workings of bioenergy relates to quantum physics, guided by <u>qualitative</u> results we have witnessed. Hopefully, the information contained herein will inspire others to develop instrumentation for accurately measuring <u>quantitatively</u> our bioenergy and the biomagnetic pairs.

According to bioenergetic basics, when disease occurs it starts at the subatomic level. Magnets somehow help the body influence that level. To see how that happens, how two magnets can help diseases such as leukemia, we need to consider other concepts. These include: pairs and duality in life, the basics of magnetism, pH and wellness, and the great variety of micro organisms and their effects on our bodies. All of these aspects enter into the art of bioenergetic basics for dynamic wellness.

CHAPTER 4
DUALITY

According to Goiz's bioenergetic model of the human body, disease can exist where our body's energy separates into two poles. When this disease-duality is absent, our energy circulates as an uninterrupted singularity. Current popular medicine as taught in most western medical schools is oblivious to this model of duality in disease formation and control. Disease is basically defined by drug- and surgery-controlled symptoms without seeking the *cause* of the disease. In his practice, Goiz has striven to show the necessity of employing simultaneously the positive and negative duality of magnetism, not limiting wellness work merely to a single polarity as is done in other magnet techniques.

Historically, the early Mesopotamians esteemed dually-entwined serpents. The ancient Mexicans believed in a supreme and dual creator OMETEOTL, called "Our Mother, Our Father" (from Miguel Leon Portilla's website, www.ejournal.unam.mx/culturanahuatl). Early civilizations also saw paired divisions in other areas of life representing them in carvings and sculptures. The yin/yang symbol of ancient China signified the divided and opposing yet complementary forces in nature. For the Chinese, there remains A principle of duality wherein yin is expansive and yang is contracting in all of existence. Acupuncture is the 2,000 year old science of balancing the yin and yang energies. In Zen Buddhism this is sometimes called "going through the gateless gate."

It is quite stupefying that conventional allopathic medicine has overlooked such a natural, simple and ubiquitous concept as duality. This oversight can be corrected by applying the principles of bioenergetic basics: depolarize biomagnetic pairs to help our body manage our wellness.

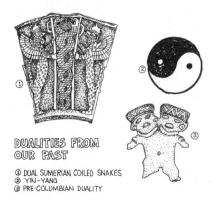

DUALITIES FROM OUR PAST

① DUAL SUMERIAN COILED SNAKES
② YIN-YANG
③ PRE-COLUMBIAN DUALITY

5. Dualities from history

1- DUAL SUMERIAN COILED SERPENTS
2- ORIENTAL YIN-YANG
3- PRE-COLUMBIAN DIETY

CHAPTER 5
MAGNETISM

Magnetism is a dual energy--one of the basic energies of matter and of the universe. Science tells us that the apparent cause of magnetism is the whirring around of electrons within atoms. Magnetism and magnetic energy have been recognized and used since antiquity.

Ancient mariners employed its energy for navigation. They would tie a magnetized lodestone to a piece of cork floating on the water. The direction it pointed would show north.

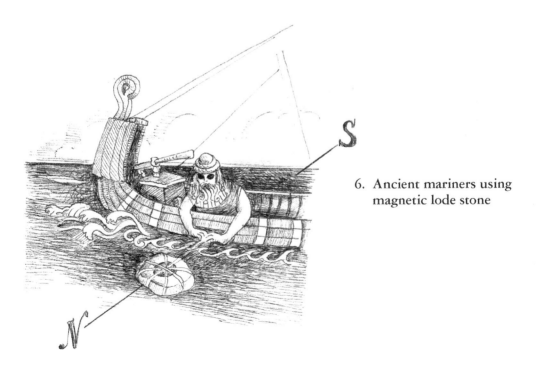

6. Ancient mariners using magnetic lode stone

In addition to its use indicating direction, magnetism's healing properties were employed thousands of years ago. Archaeologists have uncovered an ancient African mine where prehistoric miners obtained that naturally magnetized ferric compound, lodestone, known today as magnetite.

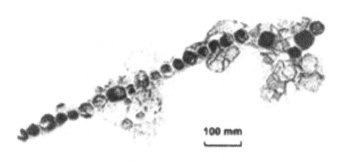

100 mm

7. Crystals of magnetite

From "Biomagnetism and Electro-Biomagnetism:
The Foundation of life in FUTURE HISTORY,
Series 1, Vol. 8, 1985, by H. Coetzee. By permission.

An ancient text from India mentions "ferromagnetic ores being used for relieving pain and acting as antidotes to poisons." (Alfredo Crossland, "New Hope Offered by Magnetic Therapies, *Journal of the Bio-Electro-Magnetics Institute* Vol. 2 No 3, fall 1990, p 7) Cleopatra and other Egyptians fastened pieces of magnetite to their foreheads supposedly to increase longevity and forestall aging. And in the Middle Ages, Paracelsus ranked the magnet as the most powerful of therapeutic agents.

Magnetism is/has a field of force. This field of force consists of two charges: negative and positive. It exists in something as small as an atom or in large bodies such as the earth or sun. Human bodies, as we stated, possess magnetic charges, as do all material things composed of atoms--plants, animals, rocks, molecules of water, etc.

Our planet is like a huge magnet. Spinning on its axis, it creates magnetic energy. The churning movement of the

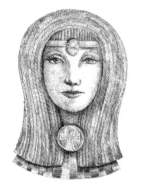

8. Cleopatra used magnetite to increase longevity

PARACELSUS

9. Magnetism was recognized as therapeutic by Paracelsus in the Middle Ages.

molten rock deep within its core produces additional magnetism. Science shows that at the earth's geographic North Pole, magnetic energy streams upward and outward. The energy can eventually circle back down towards the earth, entering at a variety of locations including at the South Pole. From the South Pole, magnetic lines also flow. The North Pole is called negative, The South Pole is positive. When speaking of energy, the title of "positive" or "negative" refers only to location (direction) of travel of energy. There is absolutely no judgment saying that positive energy is good and negative is bad.

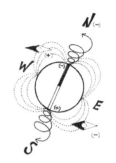

10. Earth as a magnet with North and South poles, and magnetic lines

DESCRIPTIONS OF MAGNETISM

There are certain laws of magnetism that hold true whether dealing with magnetism outside or inside of the body. One law states: **Like charges repel each other**. That means that two positive charges push against each other. Two negative ones also repel one another. A second law holds that: **Opposites attract.** Therefore, the North Pole, being negative, attracts positive charges. It also repels negative charges. The South Pole, which is positive, follows the above laws and attracts negative charges and repels positive ones.

Different conventions exist for naming magnet polarities. Physicists and certain other scientists use one definition of polarities. In bioenergetic basics, we define a magnet's negative side as "north " because it attracts the compass needle pointing north. The magnet's north side would be repelled by the North Pole, as like charges repel. The positive side of a magnet is repelled by the earth's positive South Pole while being drawn to the earth's negative North Pole. Polarities are important in bioenergetic basics as are the characteristics of attraction and repulsion--pulling and pushing. We must know when to push, when to pull; when to use positive, when to use negative (to be discussed in the section on scanning.)

The human body, mostly empty space (space within and between atoms) has tiny electrons energizing that space. When those electrons move along a path or line--like the power lines above us and nervous system within us--we call that "electricity." Acupuncture, for example, deals with energy movement along such paths or meridians and their blockages that can result in illness.

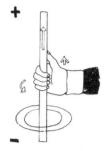

11. Hand showing flow of electrons and encircling magnetism

Magnetism is created wherever there is movement of electrons. If the electricity flows along a line, the magnetism is at right angles to the flow. Some teach that if you stick out your thumb while clenching your four fingers in toward the palm, you have created a visual aid. Your thumb represents the direction of flow of electrons. The angle between the thumb and fingers is approximately 90 degrees, the fingers showing the direction in which magnetism forms, encircling the electrical path. It is said that electrical energy (straight) seems masculine; magnetic, (curving) feminine.

Wherever there is matter, formed by atoms with their electrons in constant movement, there is magnetic energy. We have magnetic energy from elec-

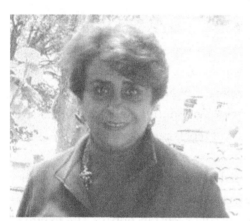

tron action within our bodies. We also contain magnetite, a ferrimagnetic mineral in the form of an intricate web involved in electromagnetic transfer throughout our bodies, as discovered in 1968 by Dr. Esther del Rio (See photo from a personal interview in autumn, 2007, at Dr. Del Rio's hacienda.)

Trauma--physical, emotional, chemical, psychological, etc.--can cause a "breakdown" to form in the normally free-flowing neutral and balanced bioenergy. Unnatural polarizations occur at those breakdowns of energy. Taking advantage of the law of magnetic attraction of opposite signs and repulsion of like signs, magnets can help locate the hidden breakdowns of energy flow in our cells, tissues, and organs. Goiz teaches that non-neutral charges manifest in the body chemistry as too many H+ ions (positive charge of acidity) and too many OH- ions (negative charge of alkalinity).

Scanning the body with a magnet can indicate these unbalanced polarized areas in our organs, tissues and cells. The biomagnetic pairs exist at the sub-atomic level of ions of H+'s and OH-'s, where diseases can start to develop before they progress to the level detectable by our five senses and by existing scientific instruments. In scanning, says Goiz,

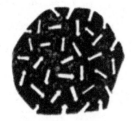 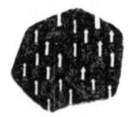

the magnet's negative pole will push against a negative area in the body. The positive magnet pole repulses a positive charge.

The atoms of non-magnetized materials can be chaotic. Once a

12. Chaotic and magnetized atoms

material is magnetized, its atoms align in a north-south direction permanently or semi-permanently. These atoms will be pulled towards the North and repelled by the South Pole of the earth, as in the illustration. This characteristic endows magnets with traits the body may use in healing itself.

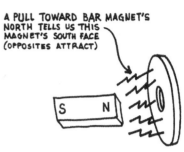

A PULL TOWARD BAR MAGNET'S NORTH TELLS US THIS MAGNET'S SOUTH FACE (OPPOSITES ATTRACT)

S   N

To work with magnets, we need to know the positive and negative sides. As mentioned, a compass will point to a magnet's negative side. If we lack a compass, we can determine which part of a magnet is north-facing by suspending it from a string. When it stops swaying, the part of the magnet pointing north is the south or positive part of the magnet, attracted by the north (negative pole of the earth). Paint the side facing north with red paint or fingernail polish so you do not forget. Once the magnet's pole is calibrated, it can then be used to identify other magnets' poles because it will either attract them or repel them.

13. Poles of a magnet attract opposite charges

Magnets have different strengths. "Gauss" is the measurement of magnetic strength, named after Johann Carl Friedrich Gauss (1777-1855), a mathematician, astronomer, and magnetism scientist. A gauss meter is the instrument that can measure the strength of the lines of magnetic flux at a specific place on the magnet.

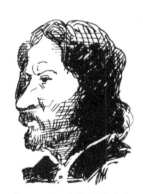

14. Johann Carl Friedrich Gauss (1777-1855)

According to magnetic engineers, a gauss reading doesn't necessarily tell what the overall strength of the magnet is. The material composing the magnet, its thickness, the date of its magnetizing, and its total size can influence its strength. Different locations on a magnet can give different gauss readings as well. There is often confusion regarding gauss but we can state that generally, "refrigerator" magnets (used for sticking doodads on the metal door) and the majority of those sold as bracelets, shoe sole inserts, pain reliever wraps for ankle, knee, shoulder, etc., and mattress pads are in the order of 700 gauss or less and lack sufficient gauss to be effective for depolarizing biomagnetic pairs. Goiz does not use them.

GAUSS OF OVER 1,000

Apparently differences in gauss measurement are not a serious drawback. Goiz is not overly concerned about the gauss of his magnets, as long as it measures at least 1,000 gauss. (A handy rule of thumb for this author is that proper magnets for depolarizing will have enough strength not to be pulled apart easily.) Goiz's reason for a seeming lack of concern about gauss is what is called the *law of all or nothing*. In the author's tapes of a lecture he gave at his clinic in April of 2002, he explained that any amount over 1,000 gauss in a magnet will make no difference in its effect upon the human body:

> *"With muscles, the <u>law of all or nothing</u> means they need a minimum electrical charge to move. More charge will just give the same muscle movement result. Less charge than sufficient will give no movement at all--nothing.*
>
> *"The same law applies to magnetic charges in biomagnetic pair work. One thousand gauss are needed. Any more gauss will do nothing more to correct the biomagnetic pair. Any less than 1,000 and there will be no permanent magnetic or polarity change.*
>
> *"You need at least 1,000 gauss to have effect. We have tested gauss from 1,000 to just below 50,000 and the result is the same. Over 50,000 and you are just getting into an amount that fatigues your body."*

> The law of all or nothing applies to biomagnetic pair work.

The power of the magnets he uses is variable as are the magnets used by the students in his clinic. As long as they fall within the range of between 1,000 and 50,000 gauss, they will be effective and non-iatrogenic (not harmful) as he has demonstrated in his practice. (Most of the magnets he uses are much less than 50,000--in the 5,000 to 35,000 range depending on the material and on how the gauss is measured).

The type of magnet he uses is what is termed a "natural" magnet. That means it keeps its magnetism naturally without having to have an electrical current constantly running through it. Natural magnets are different from non-natural or coil magnets (with electrical current) which are in use industrially, such as electron magnets used to lift heavy loads, or the high gauss magnets used in magnetic resonance imaging (MRI). As mentioned, natural magnets are not toxic and cannot produce the harmful effects derived from high power electron magnets. Such magnets are relatively inexpensive and can be obtained over the Internet or often as used magnets from electrical repair shops. Magnets from speakers and from microwave ovens are some of the ones this author uses.

> As long as a magnet's strength falls within the range of between 1,000 and 50,000 gauss, it will be effective and non-iatrogenic (not harmful). This, says Goiz, has been well-documented in his own practice.

CHAPTER 6
MAGNETIC LINES AND MIGRATIONS

The lines of magnetic energy called flux or ley lines, go around the earth and also penetrate it as well. Some ancients were more enlightened energetically than modern-day city planners, and they established sacred temples and other important buildings where the energy lines were strong. Examples would be Stonehenge, Teotihuacan and the Egyptian pyramids of Giza.

Science is now finding that certain animals such as whales, birds, butterflies, and ants, can *sense* these magnetic lines of force. (Coetzee, H., Ph.D, *Electromagnetism: The Foundation of Life, as published in Future History, Vol 8*). Other animals, including tiny one-celled bacteria, have the ability to **produce** ferromagnetic mineral crystals of magnetite (Fe_3O_4) within their bodies. With their biologically-manufactured magnetite these animals can detect the presence of magnetic lines. Using their instinctive magnetic sensitivity, they routinely navigate the great distances of their yearly migrations. (Susan A. Jungreis,"*Biomagnetism:An Orientation Mechanism in Migrating Insects?" The Flori-da Entomologist,* Vol 70, #2, p. 277.)

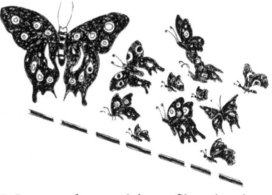

15. Swarms of monarch butterflies migrating along magnetic lines.

According to the interesting but non-scientific observations of an old Texas rancher, fire ants are aware of these lines, building their domes and super highways on them. Cows, also, seemed to him to seek out these lines just before giving birth. He often found a new born calf blinded because it had been born right on top of a line or mound of fire ants.

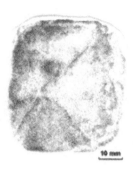

16. Crystals of magnetite from human brain tissue (from Coetzee, "Biomagnetism and Bio-Electromagnetism: The Foundation of Life, *Future History Series 1, Vol. 8, p.3*, 1985. By permission.)

Bacteria apparently detect magnetism because of the way they react to it, and can successfully orient themselves as well. In the world's oceans certain water-borne bacteria continually re-align themselves to north after the waves of the tide alter the direction they face. Goiz's work would indicate that magnetic pulling and pushing directly affects not only those ocean-borne bacteria, *but also the bacteria and viruses swimming within the waters of our own bodies.* Human-residing bacteria apparently seek negatively charged organs, tissues, or cells, due to their outer cell walls being positively charged.

Because we humans also possess magnetite in our brains, and throughout our bodies, as discovered by Dr. Esther Del Rio in 1968 (reported in Catalina Herrera's *Por las Venas Corre Luz, pp. 3-4*), we also have the potential of sensing magnetic

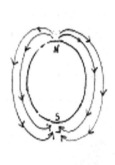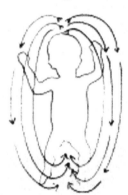

17. Our earth and our bodies with magnetic lines around and penetrating them.

energy. Perhaps we will one day discover how to put this mysterious ability to conscious use. But in order to bioenergetically manage our health, it is not necessary to develop the ability whales have to follow magnetic lines. It *is* important to bear in mind that we humans are magnetic, just as is the earth. We have magnetic charges and magnetic lines of force circling around us and through our bodies.

From studying our bodies we learn we possess a north and south pole. Goiz indicates our north pole is at our heads, the south, at our feet. Understanding this idea gets us closer to understanding how bioenergetic basics actually works just by using two magnets. Still, there remain a few other concepts such as how bacteria and viruses migrate that we must consider.

MIGRATIONS WITHIN THE BODY BY BACTERIA & VIRUSES

As mentioned, Goiz noticed a most interesting phenomenon. He found that the bacteria and viruses apparently travel within our bodies much like the migrating whales in the seas and butterflies on land. They both seem to use the same ability to home in on magnetic lines. Bacteria, equipped with magnetite particles, migrate to their preferred nesting or resting areas of our body "world". Viruses do the same. He discovered, for example, that the rabies virus consistently prefers to migrate to and "set up housekeeping" in the area of the armpits. (Rabies was the second biomagnetic pair he found). The tetanus bacteria (Clostridium tetani) migrate to the kidneys. Anthrax bacilli go to the brain.

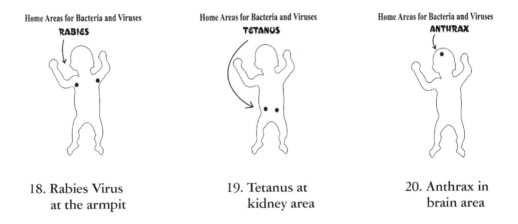

18. Rabies Virus at the armpit	19. Tetanus at kidney area	20. Anthrax in brain area

Using magnets, the doctor has located over 250 different magnetically polarized 'hideouts' of different micro organisms within our bodies. He has found that each specific condition or pathogen has manifested in the identical locations for each individual he has checked.

By identifying these prime localities in our cells, tissues, and organs, he gives anyone interested the precision tools needed for disease determination. Once pathogens are recognized (discovered with magnets), they can be eradicated or greatly weakened by the body (using the same magnets). Bioenergetic basics helps the body correct pH (acidity and alkalinity through the magnetic laws of attraction and repulsion. A correct pH is necessary for good health and for ridding the body of diseases such as leukemia. This can be accomplished by the body through the use of a simple pair of magnets.

> Using magnets, Goiz has located over 250 different magnetically polarized 'hideouts' of different micro organisms within our bodies. These 250+ points form the pairs illustrated in the section of the book entitled "Body Catalog of Biomagnetic Pairs", p. 94.

CHAPTER 7
INFLUENCES ON BIOENERGETICS

Investigations around the globe are discovering fascinating facts about our bioenergy. . Kirlian photography, for example, has indicated (and recorded) local microenvironments including temperature, pressure, moisture, etc., change our bioenergy. (Gerber, *Vibrational Medicine: New Choices for Healing Ourselves* p 54) Studies show the magnetized solar ionic particles streaming to earth from the sun, as well as the eleven year sun spot cycle, affect our health. The earth's own magnetic activity (known as geomagnetic activity or GMA) specifically influences the health of our cardiovascular system. (Stoupel, "Clinical Cosmobiology", *Newsletter of the Bio-Electro-Magnetics Institute*, p.7)

Through bioenergetic basics we can also see that geography--one's relation to the equator--also influences energy and wellness. Due somehow to magnetism of the earth and the flow of energy in our bodies, in the northern hemisphere the negative poles of the biomagnetic pairs are generally on the right side of the body. The positive poles are usually on the left side.

In the southern hemisphere it can be just the opposite. The negative halves of the biomagnetic pair often locate themselves on the left side of the body and the positive poles on the right. Goiz theorizes that the prevalence of viral versus bacterial infections is dependent on magnetism and geographical hemispheres, with more viruses originating south of the equator, more bacteria north of it, a situation meriting study, which as of yet remains inconclusive. (See Molina Pimenetel, "El Par Biomagnetico y el Hemisferio Sur," pp. 171-192)

RAINBOWS AND BIOMAGNETIC PAIRS

When a light ray traveling from the sun goes through droplets of condensation or through a prism or crystal, what happens? The condensation, prism and crystal, denser than light, act as a type of impediment, polarizing or separating the light. The white light passing through a calcite crystal divides itself into two parts. A prism divides the light into its component colors of the rainbow of the spectrum.

An important concept in bioenergetic basics is that, like light, if our bioenergy streaming around us and within us hits something powerful (a physical, psychological, or emotional trauma, etc), it can also become polarized, divided. Similar to light energy, our bio energy separates. It splits into the component parts (called positive and negative) of the biomagnetic pairs. In the presence of such abnormal charges in the body, the laws of magnetism can operate. For example, if we place a negative magnet on a negatively charged body part, there will be resistance (likes repel each other). The resistance actually occurs at the atomic level of our electrons (with negative charges). This is at that same atomic dimension where charges of pH occur and are measured and give rise to the disease-causing biomagnetic points that unite to create biomagnetic pairs in the body.

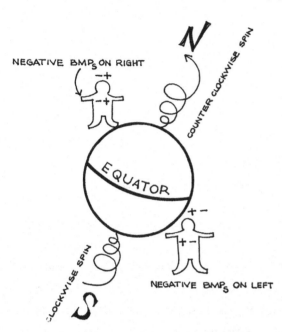

21. Charges can switch sides in different hemispheres

COMPARISON OF LIGHT ENERGY AND MAGNETIC ENERGY

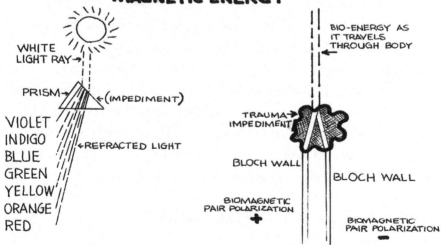

22. Light hitting a prism and a calcite crystal, and bio energy hitting a trauma, resulting in their separation.

CHAPTER 8
PH AND BIOENERGETIC BASICS

It is impossible to delve into the bioenergetic healing arts and biomagnetic pairs (BMPs) without considering the presence and influence of pH (potential or power of hydrogen). The BMPs and pH are very much a part of each other. Hydrogen, oxygen, and water are the three important components of pH which in turn affect the biomagnetic pairs. A quick review of some high school chemistry can help us to understand the model of wellness of bioenergetic basics.

HYDROGEN

The hydrogen atom is the smallest of all the atoms. The hydrogen atom is constructed of one positively charged proton in the nucleus. To perfectly balance the one positively charged proton, it has one electron. The electron has a negative charge something like an electrical spark or a wave of electrical energy. The electron buzzes around the proton much like a bee buzzing around the hive. The electron moves so fast that it produces what some scientists call the electron "cloud". They theorize that its speed causes an impenetrable electromagnetic field around the proton creating what we call matter.

Hydrogen as a component of water is very important to our body processes and health. With its single negative electrical charge, it plays a vital role in bioenergetic basics.

How does the hydrogen atom so specially relate to health and managing our bioenergy? Atoms in general and hydrogen in particular are so small that if all the nuclei of all the atoms of an entire human body were gathered together in one place, they would be no larger than a period at the end of a sentence. (Tierra, *Biomagnetic and Herbal Therapy*, p. 12). Partly due to this

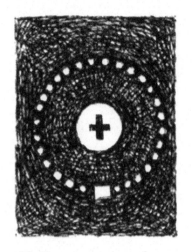

23. Representation of a hydrogen atom

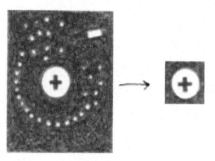

24. Hydrogen becoming a hydrogen ion (H +)

extreme smallness, the hydrogen atom can dart around very rapidly in bodily processes like a VW bug zipping in and out of 18-wheeler traffic.

A hydrogen atom can lose part of itself (its electron with the negative charge) and still function. When that occurs--if a bigger atom comes along and "shares" or "steals" hydrogen's single electron-- the hydrogen atom is no longer balanced. The little hydrogen atom without its electron becomes merely a positively charged particle (the proton that is still left in the nucleus). We call that remaining positive particle a **hydrogen ion** (or H+). This ion is a naked proton without its balancing electron clothing and it can harm our health.

The H+ is an extremely diminutive matter particle. A hydrogen ion, because of its extraordinary smallness, possesses great mobility which gives it an enormous capacity to react. Goiz indicates that with its positive charge, hydrogen can act as a *living element* in living cells. Because of this, hydrogen plays a very important role in the majority of chemical processes occurring in our body. He explains that hydrogen can also act as a *nonliving element* in our body (meaning hydrogen can enter into inorganic or non-living chemical reactions). In this inorganic capability of hydrogen, another element, oxygen, is involved.

OXYGEN

The oxygen atom is much bigger than a hydrogen atom. Oxygen has 8 negatively charged electrons that it balances with 8 positively charged protons at its center. It has two openings or vacancies in its outer electron ring for two more electrons. It "wants" to fill up the empty spaces of its outer electron ring. One oxygen molecule will "grab" on to and share the single electron of a hydrogen atom. It will actually not be completely satisfied until it attaches the electrons of <u>two</u> separate hydrogen atoms to itself to fill both of the vacancies.

WATER

When two atoms of hydrogen join with an atom of oxygen, they form a single molecule of water, H_2O. The root for the word "hydrogen" actually means "water creator" ("HYDRO" – "GEN"erator) due to what hydrogen creates in company with oxygen. Water's chemical formula can also be written "HOH" (instead of "H_2O") which can show us more clearly the association of the three atoms. Physically the two hydrogen atoms attach themselves on either side of the single oxygen atom and they can do so at different angles, forming different kinds of water.

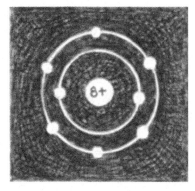

25. An atom of oxygen

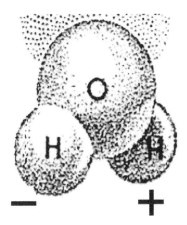

26. A water molecule

PROCESS OF ION FORMATION

Most water molecules keep their hydrogen and oxygen atoms hooked together. But every so often they can get split apart. This is one way the above-mentioned hydrogen ions can form. If the part of the hydrogen atom with the proton is knocked from a water molecule, leaving its negatively-charged electron attached to the water molecule, two things happen:

First, the separated, naked hydrogen particle becomes what we have already shown-- an ion, a charged particle due to its positive proton and its loss of the balancing negative charge (which stayed with the original water molecule). The ion is depicted as an "H" with a "+" or "H+" and is important in the study of <u>life</u> processes as it can cause chaos and imbalances at the body's energy level.

Second, the water molecule that the positive ion departed from no longer has a balanced charge either. It holds the extra unbalanced negatively-charged electron of the departed positive hydrogen ion. That extra electron gives the remaining portion of the water molecule a negative charge. It is written with an "O" for the oxygen part plus an "H" for its remaining whole hydrogen that did not get split off, plus a negative sign for the still-attached electron from the departed H+, thus "OH-". This "OH-" is called a *hydroxide anion.* Hydroxide anions are negatively-charged particles that can interfere with our wellness starting at the basic energy level.

WATER IN OUR BODIES

Our bodies are composed of a lot of water--at least 75%. This water can be neutral, positively-charged with **H+ ions**, and negatively charged with **OH- anions**. Water, whether balanced or containing excess hydroxide (OH-) anions and H+ ions, greatly influences our health. Balanced water is neutral having mostly unbroken water molecules and equal amounts of free H+ ions and OH- ions. But water's neutrality can change and become acid or alkaline. It becomes acidic when it contains many H+ ions. It turns alkaline with greater amounts of OH- anions.

In good health, the water in the body's organs and tissues is at a specific level with regard to the amount of H+ and OH-. In some organs--kidneys and stomach, for example, the body needs acidity for good health. At the same time, as in the case of blood, a slight alkalinity signals a state of well being. Hair needs a different amount of H+ and OH- than does the scalp. Saliva must differ from digestive juices in H+ and OH- content. In other words, certain H+ and OH- differences are normal within the different locations in the body.

Apparently, when these normal levels of H+ and OH- in the water in the body are compromised, pre-disease and disease states can arise at the sub-atomic level. In bioenergetic basics we seek to normalize areas of abnormal hydrogen ion and hydroxide anion levels. These abnormalities are actually points of abnormal pH or abnormal energy charges. The pH affects the activity and presence of viruses, bacteria, parasites, and fungi.

To better understand health and the workings of our biomagnetism in abating leukemia and other

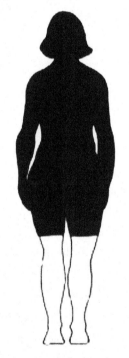

HUMAN BODY IS ¾ WATER

27. **Water content in human body**

diseases, we now turn to a discussion of pH, a clever method of measuring water's acidity and alkalinity.

pH SCALE

The 'p' of pH stands for 'potential' or 'power' The 'H' represents hydrogen. Together, they give us '**potential power of hydrogen.**' This pH scale is based on the power of 10^1. It is similar to the Richter scale for measuring earthquake intensity. The Richter scale is also based on the power of 10. Each level or gradient is ten times more powerful than the one before it.

With the pH scale, the same relationship exists. Instead of measuring the power of quakes, it rates the amount of H+ ions in water, going from 0 to 14. Neutral, in the middle, has a rating of 7 (see chart below). Less than 7 shows acidity and has progressively more H+ ions. Numbers higher than 7 indicate alkalinity and have progressively less H+ ions but progressively more OH- ions. As mentioned above, between each number in the pH scale, there is a tenfold increase or decrease in ions depending on the direction of the change. Going down (in numbers of the scale) in the direction of acidity, from 7 to 6, for example, the acidity level increases by ten times. From 6 to 5, the measured solution has 10 times more acid or H+ ions at 5 than at 6, and so on down to 1 and 0, being very, very acidic, or having a super high concentration of H+ ions.

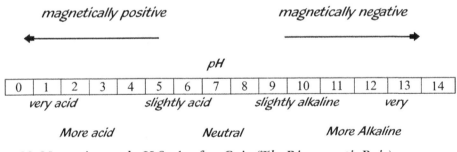

28. **Magnetism and pH Scale after Goiz** (*The Biomagnetic Pair*)

Going up numerically the opposite way on the scale, as from 7 to 8, there is an increase in the amount of OH- anions present and a decrease in the amount of H+ ions. At 8 there are ten times fewer H+ ions than at 7. This also means that there are 10 times more OH-free radicals or hydroxide anions at level 8 than at level 7. So, a pH of 8 is ten times more alkaline than one of 7. At a pH level of 9, there are ten times more OH- ions present than at level 8 and ten times fewer H+ ions, more alkalinity, and so on to 14. Level 14 is the most alkaline level of all and is the most deficient of H+ ions and has the largest amount of OH-.

All the physics and chemistry of pH depend totally on the synergy of these tiny hydrogen entities. Though infinitesimal, they powerfully influence our bodies. Because they have positive or negative charges, they can create differences in the north/south (or negative/positive) polarity of areas--cells, tissues, and organs--within our bodies. Such polarity can be observed using the north and south poles of magnets. This is what NASA's Dr. Broeringmeyer learned from studying the returning astronauts. This is what he taught and what Goiz's biomagnetic pair discovery augmented. This is also why magnets with their positive and negative poles are able to help the body influence leukemia and other diseases.

---

1) *Powers of 10*

In any amount of water, the number of H+ and OH- particles can be very great or very small. To more easily describe their amounts, science uses the powers of ten to develop a pH rating. The pH measuring system derives from a notational scale "based on counting how many times 10 must be multiplied by itself to reach a desired number. For example, 10 x 10 equals 10 to the 2ⁿᵈ power or 100. And 10 x 10 x 10 equals 10 to the 3rd power or 1000. Multiplying a number by itself gives a power of that number: 10 is read out loud as "ten to the third power" and is another way to say one thousand. In this case, there is no great advantage, but it is much easier and clearer to write or say 10 to the minus 14ᵗʰ power (which is the most alkaline) than minus 100,000,000,000,000 or one hundred trillion...." (Morrison, Philip and Phyllis Morrison and The Office of Charles and Ray Eames, POWERS OF TEN, New York: Scientific American Books, Inc,1982, p. 112)}

CHAPTER 9
EFFECTS OF ACIDITY AND ALKALINITY ON TISSUE

How do these energy or pH distortions affect the body? Goiz teaches that if the body is unable to normalize an imbalanced polarity, the affected areas become too acidic or alkaline, the start of disease. When we have an area of **hyperacidity** (low pH), there is a contraction of matter. In cases of acidic degenerative disease there will usually be no symptoms of pain. But just because there is no pain at first does not mean illness is absent. Diseased acidic areas form polarities in the body and they get smaller and harder, eventually degenerating. (See chart, p. 32)

> If there is pain,
> there is usually
> alkalinity.

Just the opposite happens in areas of alkalinity. In **hyper alkalinity** we get swelling in our body, the distention and pain of inflammation. *If there is pain, there is usually alkalinity.* Alkalinity is one reason why organs get bigger in some disease states, the presence of many OH- ions give a high pH or alkalinity with a negative charge, causing the organs to enlarge, as in the case of dysplasia.

In health, our bio energy is balanced and neutral. If we have swelling or inflammation, we have a negatively-charged area in our body. If we find shrinkage or hardness, that indicates a positive charge. The charges in these areas give us great clues about what is happening in our body and Goiz's work seems to show that the charged areas can also indicate the presence of such entities as viruses and bacteria. They can also be rated or charted, indicating the presence of leukemia and other diseases, as discussed later.

Goiz stresses the necessity of treating the actual disease at the energy level location rather than treating the area of a symptom or several symptoms. *The symptoms are not the dis-ease.* Impacting with the magnets can break up the resistance between the two parts of the biomagnetic pair (BMP). It also cancels the charges between the pair, and the energy can return to the dynamic energy level where it can flow freely once again. This is one of the differences between Goiz' method and that taught by Broeringmeyer. Broeringmeyer

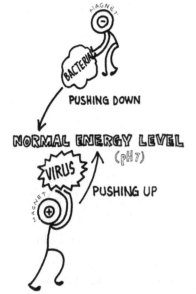

suggested putting a magnet on for 30 days to obtain results--to draw out the charges.

In Goiz's model, instead of drawing out the charges, he puts a magnetic charge similar to the one in the polarized organ(s). That allows the body to dissipate unhealthy charges and force the energy and organs back to their neutral and healthy state. That is apparently what is occurring: a positive charge placed on a positive pathological element pushes its charge up (in pH) from acidity to neutral. A negative charge pushes the high negative charge down (in pH) from alkalinity and back to the mid pH range of our dynamic wellness level of energy.

When asked what happens to a magnet during this

29. Positive magnet pushing virus up in pH; negative one pushing bacteria down

pushing of charges (often the magnets get warm or damp) Goiz has answered,

"Nothing! The magnet is only pushing charges. Magnets do not have intelligence. They only have polarity. They heat up or become damp because of the increased circulation in the tissues under them and this causes absolutely no problem."

ACIDITY   ALKALINITY

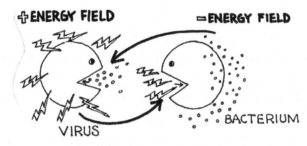

30. Two kinds of energies feeding one another

According to Goiz, both the positive and negative poles of the biomagnetic pairs "feed" each other energetically. Occasionally the positive one resonates or feeds two or more negative poles similar to how a stallion can pair with several mares.

The positive polarity pole has the more concentrated energy of the two. The negative poles are more dispersed or broader. Just as the ovum (female egg) is much greater in size than the male sperm, the negative pole of the BMP is larger than the positive one. Because the negative pole is larger, it is easier to locate within the body. For that reason, the use of the negative magnet in scanning is the easier way. We will show more on this later.

We know that usually negatively and positively magnetized objects, being opposites, attract each other. Yet in the case of the polarization of bioenergy, the separated parts seem to resist each other. What keeps the oppositely charged parts separated when a basic law of magnetism says that opposites attract?

There is an energy phenomenon in magnetism called the Bloch wall, named after the physicist Felix Bloch. A Bloch wall, according to physicists, is built up from the spin of mobile electrons, and is a narrow transition region at the boundary between magnetic domains, over which the magnetization changes from its value in one domain to that in the next. It forms a neutral center force element or neutral field. *(from Anti Gravity and the World Grid, ed. By David Hatcher Childress, Adventures Unlimited Press, pp. 64-5)* As mentioned, in Zen Buddhism this neutral central area is sometimes referred to as the "gateless gate."

Apparently when a biomagnetic pair forms there is something like the neutral Bloch wall or gateless gate in between the pair, keeping them separated. Goiz calls the area between the charged pair—within the Bloch wall—the normal energy level, the level needed for dynamic wellness.

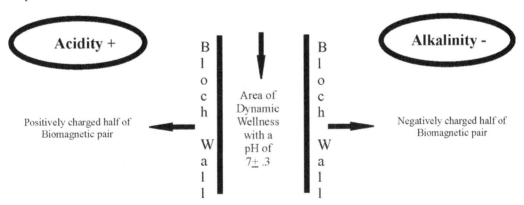

31. **Dynamic Wellness area between Bloch Walls of Polarization**

This central area of dynamic wellness is a significant place between opposites. Physicists have found that at this meeting point of positive and negative, gravity is affected. Scientists are apparently working on using that special point for "beaming" into space or even for studying other dimensions. <small>(David Hatcher Childress, ed. *Anti-Gravity & The World Grid*, p.64.)</small>

In health, the area of dynamic wellness is where all cellular metabolism happens. It is the ideal healthy place to be--centered. It is the point of unity, what might be called the Tao of our unencumbered, free-flowing energy. This space, as quantified by the pH scale as we have mentioned, is usually very close to 7 with only a '+ .3' or a ' - .3' variation tolerance. *(Goiz, The Biomagnetic Pair, p. 47)* The Bloch wall is a natural barrier which, in cases of disease, keeps the charges apart and thus keeps the disease process going. It is an insulator keeping opposite charges apart for the stability and formation of each biomagnetic pair, since opposite charges are normally attracted strongly to one another.

The following chart is based on one from Goiz's *The Biomagnetic Pair,*(*p. 51.*) It shows the two poles of diseases, positive/negative or acidic/alkaline. The positive side is where viruses and fungi appear. That side is asymptomatic at first, but finally shows degeneration of tissue.

The negative side is where bacteria and also parasites congregate. The negative side gives clinical symptoms right away, later resulting also in tissue degeneration. As explained above, even though the two poles each result finally in tissue degeneration, that degeneration is different at each pole. At the positive pole, the tissue is much shrunken. At the negative one, it is much expanded.

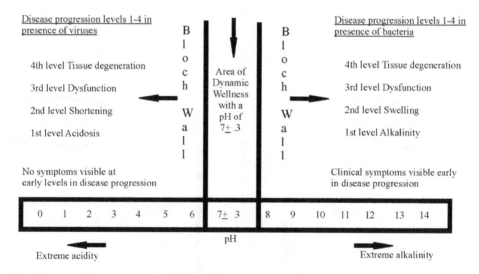

32. Disease Progression outside of Dynamic Wellness Area according to Goiz

The straight arrows pointing away from the dynamic wellness area indicate what happens when the pH becomes extremely acidic or extremely alkaline. There can be at least 4 levels in the disease progression based on pH abnormalities. When we place magnets on the biomagnetic pairs and push their polarized energies back to the center within the Bloch walls, the two sides reunite in the balance of dynamic wellness.

To further summarize, this is Goiz's model of how diseases progress on each side of the dynamic wellness area:

At the positive pole,

1. Acidosis is established in the affected organ.
2. Matter or tissue contracts or foreshortens.
3. The organ or tissue decreases in size.
4. The organ or tissue dysfunctions.
5. *Degeneration occurs.*

All five events are in the presence of a virus.

At the negative pole,

1. Alkalosis is established in the organ or tissue supporting the alkalinity.
2. Distention of matter or tissue occurs.
3. Edema and inflammation happen.
4. Organ dysfunction takes place.
5. *Degeneration occurs.*

All five occurrences are in the presence of bacteria.

As we can see, the two processes at the two poles end up with the same final result:

Degeneration. (Goiz, *The Biomagnetic Pair*, p.49)

In *The Biomagnetic Pair*, p. 15-6 Goiz declares:

"These days, the presence of free radicals is accepted and also polarization of tissues. But the phenomenon is considered as being isolated as if each polarized focus were independent and did not have a relation to the charges of the opposite sign. Dr. Broeringmeyer did not realize that there exist two biomagnetic charges in resonance, a biomagnetic pair that identifies pathology of living organisms.

"The concept of biomagnetic pairs revolutionizes all the physiopathological theories upon understanding that viral and bacterial sicknesses are in strict relationship and that the first are reciprocal with the second ones and are simultaneous in their genesis as well as in their morbid presence as well as in their final consequences. That is the irreversible degenerative process."

Theorizing as to why this polarization can happen, Goiz continues,

> *"We still do not understand -- and when we do, sicknesses will be finished--why a whole organ gets polarized in one instant, towards the positive side with an excess of hydrogen ions, falling to a state of acidity in its totality, which in turn, conditions as a necessarily logical consequence, the polarization of another organ in the opposite sign, i.e., towards alkalinity, due to a deficit of hydrogen ions and a presence of free complex radicals of negative polarity.*

> *"As we now know, hydrogen is the principle glue of organic matter. It constitutes the strongest union of the molecules. Also, from the kinetic point of view, it is the rack and pinion uniting the atoms of carbon, oxygen, nitrogen and all the other components of organic substance {It can do this} since it acts simultaneously electro negatively when it is an element and electro positively when it is an ion. All of that depends on the dynamism of the energetic shadow known to us as "electron."*
> *(Goiz, The Biomagnetic Pair, p.48)*

INTENSITY AND FREQUENCY

Goiz presents a theory about the intensity and frequency of the charge in the polarized areas. The theory holds that the opposing poles display the same charge intensity and frequency due to and indicated by the fact that they paired. He declares:

> ... *"in theory both poles present the same intensity of charge, the same biomagnetic frequency, which I have been able to prove practically since it is not possible to inhibit the pole of one B(iomagnetic)M(agnetic)P(air) with that of another pair, i.e., each . . . can be deactivated by pushing its charges internally one against another, but not that of one pair against another pair."*
> *(Goiz, The Biomagnetic Pair, p. 49)*

In other words the two points making up the biomagnetic pair are in harmonic vibration and can be depolarized by putting magnets on each one of them. The BMPs are independently depolarized even though it is possible to depolarize more than one pair simultaneously.

> The two points making up a biomagnetic pair have the same intensity and frequency.

CHAPTER 10
MICRO ORGANISMS

Goiz postulates that when disease-causing bacteria appear in the body, they gravitate to a specific location. They will wait there, he says, until they make contact with a virus of the same resonance and vibration. When that meeting occurs, the disease process can begin. Sort of like an opera diva arriving at the theater but waiting off stage until the orchestra tunes up and is at the correct pitch for her performance. The singer won't perform under any other condition.

If the virus necessary to resonate with the bacterium is not present or does not resonate in harmony, the bacterium will simply wait and there will be no duet (no disease). The disease-causing bacterium will not perform, will not produce disease. It will be latent and there will be no symptoms. It can lie patiently in waiting, even for long periods of time before making an actual appearance.

Similarly, viruses showing up in the body will not become pathological until or unless they can pair with bacteria of the same vibration with which they resonate. If that specific bacterium is absent, the virus will not produce a disease. This, explains Goiz, is one reason why some people can be exposed to the HIV virus and not get ill. They lack the corresponding bacteria needed to vibrate and resonate with the virus. The virus is impotent without its polarizing partner; *everything happens in pairs.*

When conditions exist for this resonance to occur, there is an immediate polarization of a biomagnetic pair. The bacterial partner of the pair, with its positively charged outer cell membrane, surrounds itself in negative polarity, existing in and/or creating alkalinity. The negatively charged viral part is in the positive polarity and provokes and/or needs acidity to thrive. The question as to which comes first, the bacteria or the alkalinity, the virus or the low pH, is, at this point, an unanswered "Which came first, the chicken or the egg?" question.

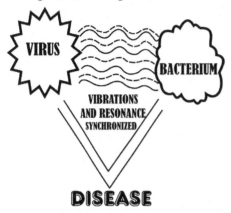

33. **Virus and bacterium resonating in harmony to produce disease**

A virus won't live in acidity without a corresponding resonance from a bacterium in alkalinity. The bacteria can't be provoking diseases in an alkaline pH without a corresponding virus of equal vibrations and resonance in its own acidic pH environment.

It is obvious that to create a baby, for example, we need both feminine and masculine energies. Likewise, to create an illness requires both positive and negative energies. If we ignore this requirement, we overlook 50% of the problem. Usually only one half of the disease is recognized and receives treatment. No wonder some illnesses reoccur and can go on seemingly indefinitely

MORE ON VIRUSES, BACTERIA, FUNGI & PARASITES

Viruses act as ions when resonating with bacteria because of their charge and tiny size. Impacting the viruses with a magnetic field of over 1000 gauss affects them *violently*. They lose their pathogenic capacities almost immediately. Their viral effects--toxicities due to their presence--reduce in critically short time periods, often in minutes or hours. Depolarizing a virus seems to destroy the virus memory, similar to what happens to a recorded

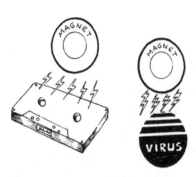

34. **Memory of cassette tape and virus being erased**

electromagnetic tape when you put a magnet on it. The prerecorded messages are erased, wiped clean. Likewise with a virus, its memory is obliterated so it no longer has an identity. It no longer **IS**. It no longer *exists* as a virus at the energy level. That is a simplistic but descriptive explanation. The bioenergetic basics method is extremely effective against viruses especially if you treat them in their beginning stage (before ensuing toxic and structural side effects can be provoked) so the body can heal itself most easily and completely.

The magnetic impacting will only allow the body to affect the active viruses at an *energetic* level. What, then, about damage on the structural, physical body? Degeneration caused on a structural level (pH and/or micro organism damage) is not affected so dramatically by magnets.. Once the damage is structural, the effects of magnets will be mostly palliative or beneficial in the healing process (but must be left in place for longer time periods, a process different from that involving biomagnetic pairs as considered in this writing). Goiz recommends routine checks to catch and prevent harmful, irreversible tissue damage from polarity imbalances and micro organism damage **before** they become structural. As such, bioenergetic basics offers an effective preventative alternative.

Bacteria are more complicated, being unicellular living entities not directly destroyed by natural magnets. They "group and sustain themselves in their metabolism, organizing themselves so as to be more aggressive."(*Goiz, The Biomagnetic Pair, p. 130*) They thrive in an alkaline environment. With magnetic energy, the body may rid itself of bacteria by radically altering their surroundings. If hyper-alkalinity is returned to a neutral pH, bacteria cannot thrive. By reducing their vigor and number, the body's own immune system has a better chance to overpower them. If the virus with which they resonate is exterminated, the bacteria lose their resonating accomplice and their shared private energy vortex. They lose their partner in crime and cease their destruction.

If there is a pathogenic bacterium present at the time of scanning and treatment, Goiz prescribes an antibiotic for the patient to take for a few days to insure that the bacteria die off quickly. He uses antibiotics as a safety net to catch any that might have survived the magnetic impacting. Alternative natural products such as herbs with antibacterial properties (garlic, grapefruit seed extract, echinacea, myrrh, etc.) may also serve in the same way.

The bioenergetic basics method deals with both members of the pair. With conventional allopathic methods, when someone is treated with antibiotics, s/he is receiving treatment for only one half of the problem (the bacteria). The viral half of the disease stays in the system, waiting for the bacteria to reappear again. Re-infection can happen much more easily. <u>By eliminating the viral partner of the pair and making it inhospitable for a bacterium, there is much less likelihood of re-infection.</u> Also, Goiz has determined that, apparently, once he magnetically impacts a bacterium, it weakens its defense mechanism against antibiotics making it more easily destroyed by antibiotics or herbal antibacterial preparations.

Goiz explains how viruses and bacteria join together in the body to form the biomagnetic pair. (See chart #36) The **virus** can be of two different types. It can be an RNA type or a DNA type. The DNA type is pathogenic, disease-causing. Whenever there is a *pathogenic DNA virus*, the bacterium of its BMP is not disease-causing. In such a pair, the *virus* causes the sickness.

BACTERIA	VIRUSES
Can live for weeks; they breathe and have a metabolism	Have ½ life of minutes; they do not breathe and do not have a metabolism
Often evolve or mutate, making lab tests and drugs ineffective	DNA (disease-causing) viruses have chain of DNA and a coat of mucoprotein. RNA viruses only support pathogenic bacteria and have no DNA..
Cancers are bacteria-related, as Goiz discovered	Goiz also found cancers have at least one viral component
Pain and inflammation are related to bacteria	If there is a virus, the body will make antigens, which provoke toxins, which can also cause an allergic reaction in the body. Viruses also produce cellular and axonal (nerve cell) irritations through body immune system reaction to them
Bacteria can be of different sizes. Their cellular structure is very different from that of the cells of the human body.	Viruses can have different weights. Insulin has a heavy molecular weight. When a virus weighs more than insulin, it does not enter into the disease process. If it weighs less, it can enter a cell easily and provoke disease.
Bacteria thrive in an alkaline, or negative environment due to the positive charge of their exterior cell membranes	A virus is negative in charge, and associates with acidity, which is of a positive charge (opposite charges attract).
With the presence of a parasite, check for the underlying bacteria, as parasites can live off bacteria	If there is mycosis (disease caused by a fungus), check for the presence of a pathogenic virus. For example, oral Candida albicans is generally supported by a virus. Get rid of the virus to deprive the fungus of its support.

35. Comparison of Bacteria and Viruses

On the other hand, when the virus is of the RNA type (non-pathogenic) then the *bacterium* of the pair is pathogenic. In that case, the virus only lends support to the bacterium, vibrating and resonating with it to strengthen it. The *bacterium* causes the disease and ensuing pain.

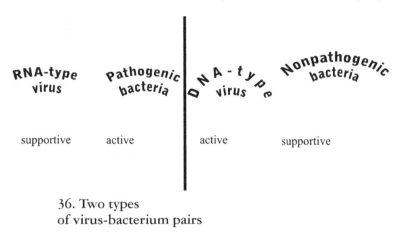

36. Two types
of virus-bacterium pairs

FUNGI, PARASITES AND BY-PRODUCTS

The art of bioenergetic basics deals with other micro organisms besides viruses and bacteria. Fungi and parasites may also be controlled by the body when using magnets. Fungi need four conditions in order to exist in the body: 1) organic matter; 2) humidity; 3) partial darkness; and 4) acid pH. The first three are part of the body normally. The fourth is made available by the presence of viruses. (See chart below) This, Goiz says, is why so many fungal diseases remain untreatable in regular medical practice. The medical practitioners do not identify the underlying virus that supports the fungus so neither an oral nor local drug works effectively. Seeking and eliminating the virus, first, and then changing the local pH to eliminate the fungus is more efficient.

Parasites, on the other hand, "can only exist in organisms where bacteria that feed them also exist in an area of heightened alkalinity." *(Goiz's El Par Biomagnetico, p.132)* To eliminate the parasites, it is first helpful to locate and destroy the bacteria that support them. Otherwise, getting rid of only the parasites will not bring lasting results, as the milieu is still favorable to parasite habitation as long as bacteria are present as their food supply.

ACIDITY	ALKALINITY
Presence of virus	Presence of bacterium
Pathogenic fungus	Parasite

37. Relationship of Virus/Fungus and Bacterium/Parasite

This chart shows Goiz's findings about the relationship of fungi with viruses and parasites with bacteria. He has found that fungi seek acidity and also live off of viruses. Parasites dwell in alkalinity and survive on bacteria and/or free radicals, which also dwell in alkalinity. <u>Therefore, when we do a scan and locate a fungus or a parasite, we need to check to find the virus or bacterium that was helping it to survive</u>. Also, if a bacterium or virus is found during scanning, the whole body should be scanned to uncover any associated fungi, parasites or other micro organisms. Often the fungus or parasite can hide or screen out a virus or bacterium in the scanning process if the fungus or parasite is very aggressive. Depending on the aggressiveness of the fungus, Goiz might use antifungal preparations in combination with the magnets.

CHAPTER 11
BIOMAGNETIC PAIRS

As mentioned, Goiz has found that the BMPs form in distortions of pH. Whatever makes the body abandon its dynamic wellness energy level of pH (7 +/- .3) gives us bio-energetic imbalance, disease. We know that in the human body, magnetic fields exist. A variation or compensation within the organism can produce a change in those fields. Those changed fields indicate the BMPs. In notes taken at Goiz's 2000 seminar, he classified the BMPs in the following five groups:

1. Regular BMPs
2. Special BMPs
3. Glandular dysfunction BMPs
4. Associated BMPs
5. Temporary BMPs

The <u>regular biomagnetic pairs</u> are the most numerous. They are formed by a combination of a bacterium and a virus, in which only the pathogenic micro organism is named.

The <u>special biomagnetic pairs</u> have titles (names of persons) in addition to names for location in the body. They are different from the regular pairs in that viruses and bacteria do not support them, except possibly for the pair named Duran. They produce cerebral, pulmonary, or renal symptoms. The Duran pair appears similar to HIV 1, but after many years of observing it, Goiz still has not identified the virus or bacteria connected with it. He thinks these special pairs are probably involved with glandular dysfunction or nerve plexus networks. There are at least 20 of these special pairs.

The <u>glandular dysfunction</u> BMPs involve various glands in the body. They cause biomagnetic pairs to originate due to circumstances other than viral or bacterial. There are 12 of them.

<u>Associated biomagnetic pairs</u> occur where various pairs unite together. They are found in syndromes such as Alzheimer's and cancer. In Alzheimer's, the BMPs Wrist/Wrist and Calcaneus/Calcaneus are both polarized. For cancer, Scapula/Scapula plus three other BMPs must be associated.

<u>Temporary pairs</u> are formed by trauma or intoxication. They spontaneously disappear when the damage is corrected. There can be an infinite number of them based on the variety of possible injuries, intoxicants or poisons. For example, heavy metal poisoning may be addressed with Pancreas/Pancreas, or pesticide poisoning with Quadriceps/Quadriceps. An injury may be helped with a negative magnet on the injury, a positive one on the kidney of the same side of the body.

In this book, the regular BMPs, the special BMPs, the associated BMPs and the glandular dysfuntioning BMPs can be found in the Body Catalog section, and in the Alphabetical List of Conditions.

GLANDULAR DYSFUNCTION BMPs

Goiz has found that often a glandular dysfunction originates not in the gland itself, but in a broader area surrounding the gland. By priming the body with magnets so it may eliminate other BMPs close to the gland, often the gland returns to normal function. For example, diagram 38 shows three additional BMPs around the thyroid besides that of Thyroid/Thyroid which could alter its function: Nasal Sinus/Nasal Sinus, Mandible/Mandible and Armpit/Armpit. At times, they could impinge on the thyroid, afflicting it. Depolarizing them, as well as Thyroid/Thyroid may be necessary for the body to achieve complete wellness.

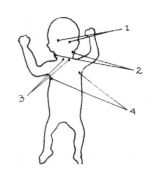

38. **BMPs afflicting thyroid**

1- NASAL SINUS/NASAL SINUS
2- MANDIBLE/MANDIBLE
3- THYROID/THYROID
4- ARMPIT/ARMPIT

ASSOCIATED BIOMAGNETIC PAIRS (BMPs)

The associated BMPs, as mentioned, create syndromes and other more complicated disease states. The body may heal abscesses, cysts and dysplasia successfully by depolarizing the contributing BMPs. The chart below (from a seminar in 2000) summarizes certain associated BMPs that yield those conditions:

1) If you find a BMP that has pathogenic bacteria associated with another BMP pathogenic bacteria, they may produce an <u>abscess</u>. Two pathogenic bacteria together may produce a <u>slow-forming abscess.</u>.

2) Two pathogenic bacteria pairs plus a fungus, may lead to a <u>fast-growing abscess</u>.

3) If there is a pathogenic virus BMP along with a pathogenic bacteria BMP, your body may form a <u>cyst</u>.

If you add to that cyst another pathogenic bacteria BMP, you may have a <u>dysplasia</u> (abnormal growth or development). An example of dysplasia is: *Borrelia* + *Vibrio cholera* + a virus = an enlarged colon. (This would show up during a scanning session as the following BMPs: Costal/Liver to hepatic duct [*Borrelia*] +Colon, Transverse/Bladder [*Vibrio cholera bacteria*] + [*Coxsackie intestinal virus*] Mango/Mango).

1 BMP pathogenic bacteria + BMP pathogenic bacteria	= *ABSCESS, slow forming*
2 BMP pathogenic bacteria + BMP pathogenic bacteria + Fungus	= *ABSCESS, fast growing*
3. BMP pathogenic virus + BMP pathogenic bacteria	= *CYST*
4. BMP pathogenic virus + BMP pathogenic bacteria + BMP pathogenic Bacteria	= *DYSPLASIA (abnormal growth or development)*

39. How Abscesses, Cysts and Dysplasia form

CANCERS AND TUMORS

Goiz owes his phenomenal success with cancers and tumors (over 10,000 cases to date, according to his estimates) to his understanding of associated BMPs. His findings, as delineated in the chart below, **show that benign tumors** occur when there are three pathogenic bacteria BMPs in combination with a pathogenic (DNA) virus. An example would be: *Actimomises bacter* (Bursa/Bursa-p.99) plus *Bordatella bacteria* (Countercaecum/Countrcaecum-p.109) plus *Escherichia coli bacteria* (Index Finger/Index Finger-p.122) plus *Enterovirus* (Malar/Sternum-p.130) coming together to create a benign tumor.

1. BMP Pathogenic Bacteria + BMP Pathogenic Bacteria +
   BMP Pathogenic Bacteria+ BMP with DNA Virus   = **BENIGN TUMOR**

2. BENIGN TUMOR + *Mycobacterium lepra* (Leprosy)   = **CANCER**, true,
                                                          with anaerobic
                                                          metatasis

40. How Benign and Malignant Tumors form

Malignant tumors, Goiz teaches, can arise from a benign tumor in the presence of Mycobacterium lepra (the leprosy cause). Most English-speaking people are not aware of how invasive leprosy has become. Goiz says he has found it present at the energy level in *every* case of malignant tumors he has treated. Leprosy is simple for the body to eradicate, putting magnets on Scapula/Scapula. With Mycobacterium lepra, even in very low levels, comes true cancer, having anaerobic (no oxygen) metastasis. He calls *Mycobacterium lepra* the "factor of malignancy," and the body must destroy it to eliminate malignancies.

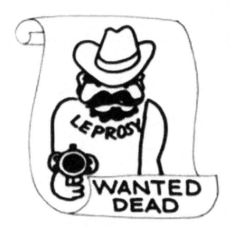

41. *Mycobacterium lepra* as criminal in
malignant cancers.

The implications of these findings are revolutionary and liberating. They need to be taught to every man, woman, and child. Every doctor and nurse, every patient suffering from cancer needs to realize this: that by aiding the body to get rid of *Mycobacterium lepra* in the early stages, true cancer may be stopped dead in its tracks by the body.

Whether a tumor is benign or malignant, its location is determined by <u>bacteria,</u> with the tumors obeying what Goiz terms a *regional bacterial factor.* Examples would be patients with leprosy and BMP Parietal/Middle Intestine (*Entamoeba histolytic*) getting tumors in the brain due to the parietal aspect of the pair. Or, a patient with leprosy and *Staphylococcus aureus* (located in the pancreas) could get pancreatic cancer. A patient with leprosy plus the BMP Humerus/Humerus (*Enterobacter pneumonia*) would be likely to get a tumor in the humerus bone. The BMP of aspergillus (a fungus), Canthus/Canthus (at the outer corner of the eye) could cause eye cancer. The cancer will appear wherever the negative pole of the bacteria is located if the cancer process is allowed to continue from the energy level forward without bioenergetic or other intervention.

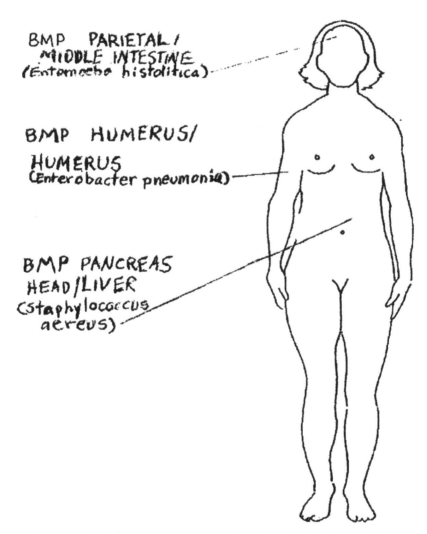

BMP PARIETAL /
MIDDLE INTESTINE
(Entomoeba histolitica)

BMP HUMERUS/
HUMERUS
(Enterobacter pneumonia)

BMP PANCREAS
HEAD/LIVER
(Staphylococcus
aereus)

MEANING THAT BY KNOWING WHERE THE
BMP IS LOCATED, THE ACTUAL SITING OF A FUTURE
CANCER TUMOR CAN BE PREDICTED.)

42. Regional Bacteria Factor of Location and Prevention of Tumors

Being able to predict the location of a cancer in the body removes much of its morbid mystique. What we strive for with bioenergetic basics is never to allow the cancer process to reach deformity on the physical level. If cancer has proceeded to materialize, bioenergetic basics still offers the body the opportunity to destroy the cancer. Utilizing the BMP knowledge may prevent or eradicate many cancers, *but not all*. Success can occur only if the growth of the cancer stops *before* permanent structural damage has occurred. Thus we can see the value of frequent and regular biomagnetic scans so as to catch and dispatch disease at the *energy* level.

By depolarizing early, the future cancerous tumor could be eliminated by the body!

CHAPTER 12
SYMPTOMOLOGY

"We are not interested in symptoms!"
-Isaac Goiz

In conventional forms of treatment where biomagnetic pairs are not taken into consideration, most doctors or therapists base their work on symptoms. They study them, describe them, catalogue them and then they prescribe the indicated treatment or medication to deal with the symptoms.

In bioenergetic work based on the BMP and pH, we don't kowtow to symptoms. In fact, by using bioenergetic basics soon enough, symptoms need never appear. Goiz does ask his patients to fill out forms listing their symptoms while giving permission for treatment. If we go by symptoms alone, we will be leaving out half of the possible disease conditions. Symptoms show up earlier where alkalinity (negative polarity) exists. The symptoms that are provoked by acidity or low pH are not going to be visible as symptoms until later stages of disease. And very often, diagnosis by symptomology is misleading, as the same symptom can be caused by a variety of situations. These can be confusing when not applying bioenergetic basics.

To reiterate, we need to scan for *both* positive and negative--acidic and alkaline. If we locate only one of the poles, we are ignoring one half of the illness. Both polarities must be located, verified, and depolarized. That can be accomplished by using both negative and positive magnets. *With bioenergetic basics what matters is the **cause** of the disease (the etiology), not its **symptoms,** which only appear later on the grosser material plane.*

As Goiz says, "Symptoms have nothing to do with etiology, the cause of illness." Symptoms arise late in the disease process. With the BMPs, disease may be identified and halted by the body before major symptoms occur. This is the ideal method for health. It is like seeing water seeping out of a teeny, tiny crack in a dam (little, almost unnoticeable problems on our energy level), and stopping the progression of the problem before it becomes a gaping hole with water gushing out (or a visible disease with symptoms and rampant destruction and degeneration).

One anecdote that Goiz tells about symptoms causing confusion or not showing up at all is that of a patient of one of his colleagues in conventional medicine during Goiz's early days of BMP research. The patient's lab work kept coming back showing only the presence of high acidity, so the colleague kept giving him more and more medication to reduce the acidity. The patient did not recover. When the colleague confided in Goiz about the difficult situation, Goiz suspected that the patient had more than only the visible disease showing up in lab reports. Distraught at losing his patient, the doctor commented to Goiz that he did not understand how he could have died when he was treating the disease "according to the book." Goiz took advantage of the opportunity to explain about biomagnetic pairing and symptoms.

He showed the other doctor that in the case of that patient, according to the biomagnetic pairs, there was not just one thing needing to be treated. Two things were going on at once. There was acidity, as the lab reports indicated. But in another part of the body there was an equally great alkalinity which did not show up in the tests. By treating only the hyperacidity, his patient died from the powerful alkaline state in the other organ that was overlooked and worsened by the medication prescribed.

In Goiz's words,

> "When the doctor found out about my system he understood that if. . . his patient...died of metabolic acidosis, the alkaline focus was also present but it was not discovered and was not freed. That occurred generally in the pancreas, i.e., if he had detected the pair and it had been impacted, the two phenomena would have been neutralized and he would not have required a single dose of carbonate." (Goiz, The Biomagnetic Pair, p. 128)

The colleague is now one of Goiz's staunchest supporters.

Goiz tells his students that a BMP is where viruses and bacteria interact. Symptoms are merely a by-product and often occur at places that are different from the BMP location. One BMP that is located at places not "logically connected" to the symptoms its micro organisms can produce is rabies. The rabies BMP is located under the left and right armpits. That is where the virus and bacteria are dealt with on the bioenergetic level. The symptoms that rabies gives usually appear in other parts of the body--larynx, ear, sinuses, thyroid, parathyroid, and parotid.

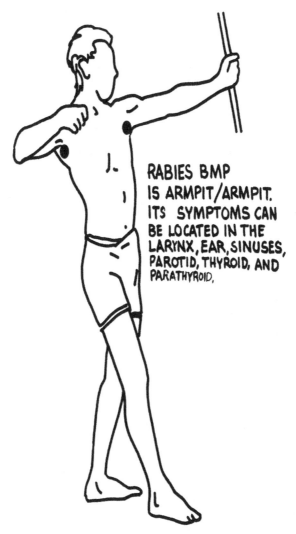

43. Rabies under arms, with symptoms in other areas.

Another element which is often not taken into account by conventional medicine is the part played by **sub products** that are created by the micro organisms. Viruses, bacteria, fungi, and parasites can all produce toxic by-products while they live as well as after they die and their bodies decompose. These toxins *"increase the symptomology or make it more diffuse, confusing and profuse....but...upon identifying the BMPs and depolarizing them {they} mitigate their production and their pathogenic manifestation."* (Goiz, *The Biomagnetic Pair, p. 133-4*) An example of this is the **ribosome** which is given off when bacteria die. If the ribosomes are excessive they become toxic and can produce bone pain. *Staphylococcus aureus magalasa+* produces toxic ribosomes and polypeptides as a result of its metabolism. They can produce a "false" rheumatism, successfully eliminated by the body after depolarizing its biomagnetic pairs.

There is a multitude of symptoms that imitate true disease states but are actually false representations often leading to misdiagnoses. These copycat diseases come about due to the presence of biomagnetic pairs or to the toxicities of by-products produced by the micro organisms and their toxins. Goiz classified an entire section of these misdiagnoses as "false positives." When patients come to him with states of disease that have been resistant to conventional medical treatment, they bring their medical records and laboratory reports which indicate the supposed disease.

In his efforts with these patients, Goiz has compiled some amazing percentages on the accuracy of their previous diagnoses. He claims that, for example, arthritis was misdiagnosed in a whopping 80% of cases. One percent of diabetes mellitus was due to pancreas dysfunction and the rest due to other causes. "Cancers" were often not cancerous, but were a combination of bacteria and viruses and as such were curable by the body with bioenergetic basics.. "AIDS patients have come to him who magnetically scan out as having no HIV but rather a totally different set of microbes that are completely treatable.

Below are some of his findings for false positives (wrong diagnoses) which mimic the real diseases. (*Goiz, The Biomagnetic Pair, pp. 136-137*) To take an example from the chart, patients have come to him with a previous diagnosis of "diabetes mellitus". As the chart indicates, he has found the presence of fifteen different micro organisms (under the column titled "possible diagnosis" from *Salmonella typhus* bacteria to *Helicobacter pilori*), located in various parts of the body (shown under the column entitled "Corresponding BMP") which may cause pancreas dysfunction. The patients with one or more of the differentially diagnosed BMPs did not necessarily have diabetes mellitus. It is a good idea to scan for these incorrectly named diseases, especially if the person's condition has not responded to conventional allopathic treatment.

CHART OF COMPARATIVE DIAGNOSIS		
DIAGNOSIS PRIOR TO SCANNING	**POSSIBLE DIAGNOSIS AFTER SCANNING**	**CORRESPONDING BMP**
Arthritis, articular and rheumatoid, rheumatism	**Treponema palidum**	Deltoid, Middle/Deltoid, Middle
	Rickettsia	Calcaneus/Calcaneus or Wrist/Wrist

	Staphylococcus aureus	Pancreas Head/Adrenals or Pericardium/Pericardium
	Viral pleuritis	Armpit/Armpit or Pleura/Pleura–two sides
	Aphthous virus	Carina/Carina
	Viral parotiditis	Pudendal/Pudendal plus Parotid/Parotid
	Dengue virus	Pituitary/Bladder or Rachidian Bulb/Bladder
	Malaria	Cheekbone/Opposite kidney
	Epstein-Barr virus	Occipital/Occipital
	Typhus virus	Temporal/Temporal or Trochanter, Major/Trochanter, Major
	Streptococcus fecalis	Cervical plexus/Cervical Plexus
Bladder problems	**Parotiditis virus**	Pudendal/Pudendal, etc Bladder nerve similar to that of internal secretion glands, and its function can be altered by toxins from various micro organism products such as histamine, properdine, polypeptides, lysozyme, urea, creatine, etc.
Diabetes mellitus (Pancreas dysfunction)	*Salmonella typhus* **bacteria**	Trochanter, Major/Trochanter, Major
	Chlamydia trachomatis	Duodenum/Left kidney
	Chlamydia pneumonia	Hip/Hip
	Trichomonas	Caecum/Caecum
	Haemophilus **influenza**	Caecum/Caecum
	Vibrio cholera	Transverse colon
	Enterobius vermicularis (Pinworm)	Pylorus/Liver
	Shigella bacteria	Achilles/Achilles
	Pasteurela bacteria	Colon, Descending/Liver
	Enterobacter cloacae	Colon, Descending/Colon, Descending
	Trypanozoma cruzi	Costodiaphragmatic/Costodiaphragmatic
	Yersinia pestis	Flank/Flank, Spleen/Spleen, Testicle/Testicle, Vagina/Vagina
	Staphylococcus dorado	Pancreas Head/Adrenals

	Helicobacter pilori	Hiatus/Right Testicle
Kidney problems	**Aspergillus fungus**	Canthus/Canthus
	Mycobacterium tuberculosis	Supraspinal/Supraspinal
Pancreas problems	**Parotiditis**	Pudendal/Pudendal or Parotid/Parotid
Parathyroid gland dysfunction		See thyroid BMPs
Parotid gland dysfunction		See thyroid BMPs
Pineal gland dysfunction	**Anthrax bacillus**	Cranial/Cranial
	Cytomegalovirus	Eye/Eye
	Dengue, common	Pituitary/Bladder
	Dengue, hemorrhagic	Rachidian Bulb/Bladder
	Exanthematique typhus virus	Temporal/Temporal
	Neisseria catarrallis	Eyelid/Eyelid
	Viral encephalitis	Parietal/Parietal
	Viral meningitis	Rachidian Bulb/Thyroid
	Citomegalovirus	Eye/Eye
	Dengue, common	Pituitary/Bladder
	Encephalitis, viral	Parietal/Parietal
	Enterovirus	Malar/Sternum
	Haemophilus influenza	Caecum/Caecum
	Meningitis, viral	Rachidian Bulb/Thyroid
	Neisseria bacteria	Mandible/Mandible and/or Eyelid/Eyelid
Spleen		See pancreas
Thyroid gland dysfunctions	**Aphthous virus**	Carina/Carina
	Balantidium typhus parasite	Cervical 3/ Supra Spinal
	Diphtheria bacillus	Subclavian/Subclavian
	Enterobacter pneumonia	Humerus/Humerus
	Herpes 2 virus	Tonsil/Tonsil
	Influenza virus	Trachea/Trachea

	Leishmania parasite	Deltoid/Kidney of same side
	Leprosy bacillus	Scapula/Scapula
	Mange or scabies	Tongue/Tongue
	Neisseria gonorrhea bacteria	Mandible/Mandible
	Pertussis bacillus	Larynx/Larynx
	Rabies virus	Armpit/Armpit
	Streptococcus fecalis	Cervical Plexus/Cervical Plexus
	Streptococcus fragilis	Angle/Angle
	Treponema palidum bacteria	Deltoid, Middle/Deltoid, Middle; also check Quadrate/Lumbar and Quadrate/Quadrate
	Tuberculosis bacillus	Supraspinal/Supraspinal
	Viral parotiditis	Pudendal/Pudendal and Parotid/Parotid
	Brucella abortus bacteria	Diaphragm/Kidney
	Candida albicans fungus	Diaphragm/Diaphragm
	Enterobacter pneumonia	Humerus/Humerus
	Escherichia coli bacteria	Index finger/Index finger
	Fasciolopsis buski parasite	Esophagus/Esophagus
	Helicobacter pilori bacteria	Hiatus/Right Testicle
	Histoplasma capsulatum fungus	Esophagus/Left side of Bladder
	Influenza virus	Trachea/Trachea
	Pleuritis virus	Armpit/Armpit, Pleura/Pleura
	Pneumocystis carini fungus	Chondral/Chondral
	Proteus mirabilis bacteria	Costal/Costal, Renal Capsule/Renal Capsule, Sacrum/Sacrum, Mediastinum, Inferior/Mediastinum, Superior
	Rubeola virus	Thymus/Left Parietal

44. Table showing misdiagnosed diseases (Goiz's false positives)

CHAPTER 13
SCANNING WITH MAGNETS

Once we understand how bioenergetic basics works, we are ready for the scanning process. Lab test results may be checked and verified with magnets. If we have an unknown malaise or merely wish to scan our body to make sure all is well, the scanning procedure gives us information about what is going on in the body. The scanning procedure actually has two parts, called by Goiz diagnosing and treating. Here are some practical hints about using magnets before putting them into bioenergetic use.

USING AND STORING MAGNETS

<u>Great care must be used when working with magnets.</u> The magnets we use are not toys. Keep them away from children, credit cards, pace makers, computer hard drives, analog tapes, and videos. They can slam together, harming fingers or pinching and injuring skin. The best way to be safe is to follow this rule: *Handle only one magnet at a time.* By handling only one magnet at a time, we are much less likely to drop one or break one, and we don't risk hurting someone.

The circular ceramic magnets like the ones used in television speakers and microwave ovens are fairly strong. If stuck together, you may not be able to pull them apart. <u>You must slide them apart instead of trying to pry them apart.</u> That will help to avoid broken fingernails or other injuries. If they are extremely hard to slide apart, try pushing one of them

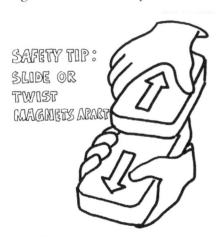

SAFETY TIP: SLIDE OR TWIST MAGNETS APART

45. How to separate magnets

against the edge of a table while sliding off the other one. Their magnetic strength can be considerable. It deserves our respect.

Using leather-, plastic-, cloth- or rubber-covered magnets can help to avoid the magnets-sticking-together situation. They are readily available on the Internet, or you can get used magnets and attach covers yourself. The author's daughter sews her magnets into socks for ease of use, to avoid loosing them, and to double as a tie to hold the magnet in place on the body (if the sock is long enough.) Some people prop the magnets in place with pieces of wood, bean bags or pillows. Various kinds of tape can also be used. With squirmy children, magnets stay in place better when the wee ones are asleep.

Exercise caution when storing magnets. Keep magnets of similar size and gauss together. Do not allow less powerful magnets to stay in contact with stronger ones, as the stronger ones can pull away the magnetic power or gauss from the weaker ones.

SCANNING Scanning is a way to discover energy polarization disturbances by placing a magnet over points on the body and checking for "short leg phenomenon." The process begins with the following steps, A-E:

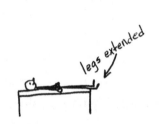

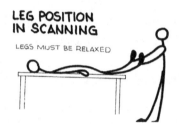

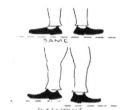

46. Position for Scanning

47. Person's legs being raised to check heels

48. Legs of same, differemt lengths

A. PERSON LIES ON BACK

Have the person to be scanned lie on her/his back with shoes on. The corners of the heels of the shoes give us two right angle edges as reference points. With bare feet and open-heeled sandals, the change in lengths of rounded heels is harder to compare, so have the person wear closed-heel shoes. The feet should hang over the edge of the table, protruding at ankle level. It is best to use a table with a firm base of a comfortable work height. It should be made of wood or some other material that is non-conducting. This avoids interference with the magnets. The person need not remove clothes as long as they are not too thick. They should be light, preferably of natural fibers such as cotton. However, Goiz scans patients who are wearing light synthetic clothing as well, and scanning has been done with the person lying on the floor if no table is available.

B. PERSON RELAXES

Have the person relax the mind and the body, arms at sides. Often it helps to have them close their eyes and block thoughts so as to focus on something calming Relaxation is very important because if there is tension, especially in the legs, the subtle changes that are used in diagnosing and treating may not be noticeable. An example of this was the author's experience in the Philippines, where the women found it very hard to relax their legs, and the scanning process had to be stopped until they could allow relaxation.

C. LENGTH OF HEEL CORNERS CHECKED

First, check visually for evenness of length of the legs by observing the heels. With your right hand holding their left leg and your left hand holding their right, raise the legs about 6 inches off the table, the feet together. Hold above the ankles so as not to touch the shoes. Move the legs apart, then together several times. Pull slightly towards yourself as you move the legs apart to make sure the knees are not bent. Legs must be suspended in air to be able to detect subtle length changes.

Make sure you are exactly centered in the front of the person so you are not pulling one leg more to one side than another. Look at the position of the left and right heels. When they come together they should be even.. If heels are even, *i.e.*, if legs are the same length, proceed to Step D below. If they are of uneven lengths, as in figure # 49, do Step E *before* doing Step D. (Some practitioners find sitting while checking leg length more user friendly than standing.)

D. SCAN BODY GOING THROUGH THE LIST OF BIOMAGNETIC POINTS IN THE BODY CATALOG SECTION OF THE BOOK (Go through the points alphabetically). Or, the points can be scanned from head to toe, referring to the diagrams preceding the title page of this book. If the BMP is bilateral, *i.e.*, Eye/Eye or Armpit/Armpit,

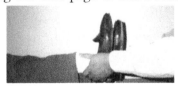

49. **Scanning, showing legs of different lengths**

you need check only one of the sides of the body. Usually, in the northern hemisphere, you check only the bilateral point on the right side of the person's body with the negative magnet. If you are in the southern hemisphere, this advice may not apply and you may need to check both parts.

Hold the magnet with negative side pointing towards the person's body. Place the negative side of the magnet at the first point you are going to check and secure the magnet. Leaving the magnet secured over the point, walk back to the person's heels. Lift the legs again and move them out and back together a few times. Check where the heels meet. If they are still the same length and meet with corners together, as before, there is no polarization or BMP at that point. Set the legs down gently. Pick up the magnet and place it on the next point to be checked. Proceed to check the next point on the list. Continue until all points are scanned, checking leg length each time.

If, after placing a magnet and when checking the heels, they are **not** even, it means you have encountered a polarized point!! If the left leg suddenly looks longer (i.e., the right leg is *shorter*), the negative magnet has hit upon the negative partner of a BMP. It produces an overcharge or energy overload from the resistance of negative against negative. It causes the right leg to shorten. There is a **biomagnetic negative pole** at that point.

(from personal seminar notes, p. 15)

> If the point happens to be on a large organ such as the liver, move the magnet around over the liver to check where exactly you get the greatest difference in heel length.

On the other hand, if in scanning with a negative magnet, you touch a point where a *lengthening* instead of a shortening of the right leg occurs, you have found where an abnormal *positive* charge in the body resides. The negative magnet pulls upon the positive partner of the biomagnetic pair and causes the right leg to lengthen. There is a **biomagnetic positive pole** at that point. Put a positive magnet there, and with another negative magnet, continue scanning.

One idea that makes the scanning go faster is to have a helper either move the magnets while you stay at the feet or vice versa to avoid having to go back and forth between the positions. Goiz has the patient or another person hold the magnet(s) in place while his assistant continues on with the scan. The magnet can also be taped or propped in place.

If the point happens to be on a large organ such as the liver, move the magnet around over the liver to check where exactly you get the *greatest* difference in heel length and place the magnet there.

Once you discover a biomagnetic point and place a negative magnet on it, you are ready to locate and place the second magnet on the second point of the pair. Proceed to chapter 14 which deals with the actual recovery part (or second magnet placement) of the scanning process.

E. DO THIS STEP ONLY IF LEGS ARE UNEVEN *BEFORE* PLACING MAGNETS

This step involves checking for the Goiz Special Biomagnetic Pair. If in doing step C (above) you find that the legs are of different lengths, you must check to see if the unevenness is caused by body structure or by bioenergy. If the difference is structural (permanent and unalterable with magnet energy), note where the two heels meet. Use that point as your reference point to gauge whether one of the leg lengths changes as you scan. You can make a mark with chalk on the side of the longer shoe or with a piece of masking tape as a secure reference. If the leg length difference is structural it is not going to be changed with magnets which work on an energy level, but bioenergy work can still be accomplished.

Likewise, if the person is missing a leg or foot, the arms can be used instead of the legs to ascertain if there are polarized areas. Instead of checking heel alignment, the corners of the thumbnails can be observed, making sure that the elbows are not bent.

If the uneven lengths are caused by an energy imbalance, then depolarizing the Goiz special pair can resolve the situation, making the legs even. The following section explains how this is done.

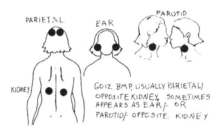

50. **Goiz Special Pair which gives difference of heel length**
until depolarized GOIZ SPECIAL PAIR

GOIZ SPECIAL PAIR

To determine whether STRUCTURE or ENERGY is causing the length difference of the legs, you need to eliminate the special BMP named Goiz as the possible cause. The Goiz special pair's biomagnetic points are located on:

a) The kidney of the same side of the body as the shortened leg

b) The second point of the Goiz special pair is in one of four areas on the opposite side of the body: <u>parietal</u> (on the upper "side edge" of the skull); <u>ear</u> (over the ear canal opening); <u>parotid</u> (under ear by corner of jaw); or <u>parathyroid</u> (under ear at thyroid height).

To clear an energy-caused shortening, do the following:

1). Reach under the patient and place the *positive side* of the magnet facing the **kidney** area on the **same side** of the body as the short leg.

2). Place the *negative side* of the other magnet on the **parietal point on the opposite side of the body**. If the short leg is on the *right*, the positive magnet goes on the *right* kidney, the negative goes on the parietal point on the *left* side. Check to see if the heels have then become even. If not, leaving the positive one on the kidney, move the negative magnet to the ear on the left side and re-check for heel evenness. Continue on to scan the parotid and parathyroid points on the left side to see if one of those points causes the leg to lengthen so both heels are even. If the *left* leg is shorter, follow the same process, placing the positive magnet on the *left* kidney and checking the four points of the Goiz special pair on the *right* side of the body.

3). If the shortening is caused energetically, the legs will become the same length with the magnets in two of these places—*the kidney and either the parietal, ear, parotid or parathyroid.* Leave the magnets in place for 25 minutes or more (longer if you live north of Mexico City or at similar latitudes south of the equator) to correct for the Goiz BMP.

With the magnets in place, proceed to Step D (above) to finish the first part of the scanning process.

A question often raised by students when scanning for the first time is: "Why does only the right half of the body lengthen or shorten with a magnet on the biomagnetic pole and not the left half? Goiz's answer is that apparently the left half of the body does not suffer such variations because the electromagnetic current of the heart beating some 80 times a minute on the body's left side keeps it more electromagnetically balanced so it doesn't shorten.

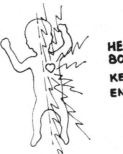

**HEART BEATING
80 TIMES/MINUTE
KEEPS BODY'S LEFT SIDE
ENERGETICALLY COHESIVE**

51. Heartbeat keeping left side normal

CHAPTER 14
BIOENERGETIC BASICS: ARTFORM TAKES SHAPE

Once a negative magnet has found its "canvas" for depolarization, it is time to bring the artistic energy creation to life. Goiz accomplishes this with a second magnet (positively charged). With the two magnets in place, the body may begin to break up the polarized biomagnetic pair. Our artistic endeavor works to achieve what great artists have struggled with throughout the ages: a reconciling of positive and negative. In this way, our fundamental bioenergy can be re-established, creating the masterpiece of dynamic wellness.

The placing of the positive magnet begins the actual performance. With the second (or positive) magnet in place, the body can push the separated charges of the biomagnetic pair across the

A DUAL TOOL

52. Biomagnetic Management as a "Dual" Tool of Discovery and Recovery.

Bloch wall. The positive and negative energy can then reunite within the bioenergy area for dynamic wellness. The formerly separated, polarized pairs cannot be reunited until **both** negative and positive charges are *simultaneously* depolarized. *The reuniting of energy of biomagnetic pairs means discovery and recovery commence. This is the beginning of wellness, the creation of this sublime energy art form.*

Goiz's discovery could prove to be one of the greatest ventures into inner space, the final frontier. The locating and identifying of biomagnetic pairs, determining their polarity, proper placing of the magnets, and subsequent depolarizing of the biomagnetic pair, are all the result of painstaking research and treatment of tens of thousands of patients, primarily in Mexico City. The hardest part of this new frontier was the cataloguing of each biomagnetic pair as they were discovered. This book contains 250 + pairs discovered by Goiz to date. Since the hard part is over (the discovery and organization), all that is left for you to do is to follow the map he has created to make your own inner space voyages and to find the hidden treasure of wellness. It's now almost as easy as painting by numbers!

Once the site of the first point of a biomagnetic pair is located,

1. **Refer to the Body Catalog** where all the points and pairs are listed alphabetically (p.132).

2. **Find the name of the second member of the biomagnetic pair.** For example, supposing the right leg shortens when negative magnet is placed on the point at the base of the neck. You look up "Neck" in the Body Catalog. On page 177 you will see two possible biomagnetic pairs under "Neck." The possible pairs are: Neck/Neck and Neck/Femur. Check first to see if the pair is Neck/Neck by placing the positive magnet at the base of the neck on the side of the body opposite to the first magnet. Check the feet to see if the positive magnet at the "Neck" position has caused the heels to become even. If the heels are even, you have hit the right spot and you know you need to depolarize the biomagnetic pair called Neck/Neck. You can see by reading further that it is the location for *Blastocystis hominis* fungus, which can go to the lungs, radiating later to the skin, bladder and prostate.

3. **If there is no change in leg length** when you place the positive magnet on the other Neck point, then Neck/Neck is **not** currently a polarized biomagnetic pair. **Return to the other possible biomagnetic pair** listed under "Neck." That pair is Neck Femur. Since there are two femurs in the body, you will need to check both the right femur and the left femur with the positive magnet. Whichever femur is polarized is the second partner in the biomagnetic pair Neck/Femur. Check with the positive magnet, placing it on each femur until you find if it is the right femur or the left femur which causes the legs to be the same length. This pair is good for helping the body be inhospitable to fungus.

4. **Leave both magnets in place for about 25 minutes.**

"Art," according to the dictionary, is human effort to supplement or alter the work of nature. The art of bioenergetic basics for dynamic wellness progresses naturally when both magnets are properly, securely and simultaneously placed. In finalizing the creative process as artists of energy, the final step is to:

Rest, stay out of the way, and let the body carry out its magnetic energy artistry.

Depending on the virulence of the micro organism destroyed through bioenergetic basics, a person may afterwards experience what some term a "healing crisis," (such as fever, vomiting, diarrhea, etc.), or natural ways the body gets rid of impurities. Goiz does not usually put much emphasis on such natural cleanses. A crisis is not usual although micro organisms in some pairs leave more pollution in the body than do others. These are noted, if applicable, in the information about each point. Goiz stresses to the patient that "the cure has been done." All that is left is for the toxins to leave and wellness to return. This may take about one week. Syndromes and stubborn, chronic situations may require more sessions depending on results.

> The art-form consists of: placing the magnets, being still, awaiting quietly. . . the marvelous healing work of the body.

HOW MAGNETS CAN BREAK UP POLARIZED BIOMAGNETIC PAIRS

PATHWAY OF NORMAL
FUNDAMENTAL BIO (LIFE) ENERGY

IMPEDIMENT→

BLOCH WALL

BLOCH WALL

POLARIZED MAGNETIC
ENERGY (+BMP IN BODY)

POLARIZED MAGNETIC
ENERGY (-BMP IN BODY)

+ MAGNET

+ BMP

- BMP

-MAGNET

POSITIVE MAGNET PUSHES
+BMP CHARGE ACROSS
BLOCH WALL BARRIER.
FUNDAMENTAL BIO ENERGY
RE ESTABLISHED.

NEGATIVE MAGNET PUSHES
-BMP CHARGE ACROSS
BLOCH WALL BARRIER.
FUNDAMENTAL BIO ENERGY
RE ESTABLISHED.

53. Magnets allowing the body to reunite
polarized BMPs, returning energy to wholeness, oneness

64

CHAPTER 15
OTHER CONSIDERATIONS

SCANNING AND RESERVOIRS

Goiz theorizes that polarized points of several biomagnetic pairs serve as reservoirs of viruses or bacteria, much like secondary refuges in the body. Once these reservoir pairs are depolarized with magnets, the bacteria and viruses taking refuge in them must flee immediately back to their primary home places. For example, if antibiotics are being taken for *Streptococcus A* (normally based in the Brachial/Brachial biomagnetic pair), the Strep A bacteria may flee to a reservoir such as Vagus/Kidney, a reservoir for viruses and bacteria. (See diagram #54) After the person stops taking antibiotics (which the bacteria perceive as a danger)--the strep could return to its Brachial/Brachial base. For that reason, reservoirs can be scanned *first* in the scanning sequence, after having checked beforehand to make sure the feet are even.

A virus reacts in a similar way. If hit by antiviral drugs or antiviral procedures, the virus can also take shelter in a reservoir. Then later it may leave the reservoir and return to home base. For this reason Goiz acknowledges his considerable respect for viruses and bacteria for their ability to act somewhat consciously to avoid detection or elimination.

Yet Goiz does not scan the reservoir pairs first. However, if he comes upon the reservoir pairs during scanning and they are "active" (or polarized, causing the leg to shorten) he must redo the entire scanning process once he has depolarized the particular reservoir pair because he can't tell exactly which micro organisms they were. Viruses and bacteria will escape to and show up at locations he may have already scanned. Scanning for reservoirs first can obviously save time and work.

RESERVOIRS:

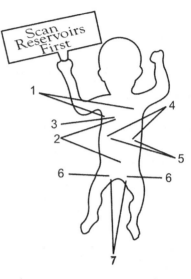

1- PLEURA/PLEURA
2- PLEURA/PERITONEUM
3- GALL BLADDER / GALL BLADDER
4- RENAL CAPSULE/RENAL CAPSULE
5- KIDNEY/RENAL CAPSULE (4 POSSIBILITIES)
6- INGUINAL NERVE/INGUINAL NERVE
7- LESSER TROCHANTER/LESSER TROCHANTER
8- VAGUS/KIDNEY (NOT SHOWN)
9- CARDIA/TEMPORAL (NOT SHOWN)
10- SUB DIAPHRAGM/SUB DIAPHRAGM (NOT SHOWN)
11- STUB/STUB (NOT SHOWN)

54. Scanning reservoirs first as an option

Descriptions of the eleven possible reservoir BMPs:

1) **Pleura/Pleura** is a possible reservoir for cancer.

2) **Pleura/Peritoneum.** Moises Special Pair. (Membranes covering inner chest and intestines, respectively) Hides bacteria.

3) **Gall Bladder/Gall Bladder.** Prada Special Pair. When broken up, the charges go to Thymus/Parietal.

4) **Renal Capsule/Renal Capsule** includes the area from the kidney almost to the scapula.

5) **Kidney/Renal Capsule** is Ale Special Pair for HIV and perhaps other viruses.

6) **Inguinal Nerve/Inguinal Nerve.** This is a reservoir for HIV 3 virus. Upon depolarization the virus goes to Thymus/Rectum.

7) **Trochanter, Lesser/Trochanter, Lesser** could be an HIV 4 reservoir...Still under observation.

8) **Vagus/Kidney** of opposite side: Benavides Special Pair. This pair is a universal reservoir of viruses and bacteria.

9) **Cardia/Temporal.** Boch Special Pair for prions.

10) **Sub Diaphragm/Sub Diaphragm.** Ecuador Special Pair for Cysticercus (pork tapeworm)

11) **Stub/Stub.** Wherever an organ or limb has been removed or incisions made, the area may harbor micro organisms. (See below)

SCANNING AND PREVIOUS SURGERY

If a person has undergone surgery, the area invaded by the knife can harbor a variety of polarizations. This can be true even long after surgery. Check all former surgery areas as well as "stumps" or "stubs" of excised organs or amputated limbs. If polarizations are present, it is likely that micro organisms have set up shop. Kirlian photography, which shows electron discharge trails around body areas similar to the corona around the sun, has shown that if a piece of a live leaf is cut away and a photo is taken of what remains of the leaf, the energy of the cut-away part is still intact. Amputees often say they can feel the energy of the limb they lost. In bioenergetic basics we have reason to believe that if a finger, for example, has been physically removed, the energy of that finger is still present.

At this point the evidence is anecdotal yet there are numerous instances of problems being removed by the body by depolarizing the residual energy of a stump or amputated limb. Any such limbs or body parts need to be scanned because their energy may contain remnants of polarized energy which may cause problems.

A common situation seen by Goiz is that of women who have had a hysterectomy, who no longer possess a uterus or cervix and may have also lost ovaries, oviducts, lymph nodes, and lymph channels. The remaining biomagnetic energy in those areas often retains previous health imbalances despite the absence of the physical organ. This explains why some women still are plagued by their original symptoms despite having suffered a hysterectomy to "correct" bleeding or pelvic inflammation. They bleed as if the uterus were still present even after its removal. Surgery could possibly be avoided with the simple, non-invasive bioenergetic basics techniques. With hysterectomies the biomagnetic pair Stub/Stub, also called Special Pair Guadalupe, requires a pair of magnets at the surgery site for the body to depolarize any existing reservoirs. In this case it would also be wise to scan the body for Uterus/Uterus as well as Vagina/Vagina and Fallopian Tube/Fallopian Tube.

EFFECTS OF IMBALANCED POLARIZED ENERGY OF MALE AND FEMALE REPRODUCTIVE ORGANS

In another example, a woman's problem may exist at the energy area of the BMPs normally associated only with males. Penis/Penis, Prostate/Prostate and Testicle/Testicle can be negatively affected in a woman as well as in a man. Ridding her of polarities in the area of masculine gender organs can rid her of previous seemingly unsolvable problems such as excessive facial hair, acne and menstrual difficulties. This is also possible with males, but reversed, with involvement for them of Uterus/Uterus, Vagina/Vagina, Ovary/Ovary and Fallopian Tube/Fallopian Tube. How can that be?

From the time of conception forward into adulthood, each person carries gender energy and possibilities of both sexes. In a female, the masculine pairs are dormant. But they still appear to be present at the bioenergy level. Likewise in a male, the uterus, vagina, and fallopian tube energies exist from conception. Although it may seem odd, scanning someone of either gender should include *both* feminine and masculine reproductive organs. Though not developed on a physically observable plane, they do exist energetically and can harbor polarizations and micro organism reservoirs. This has been demonstrable through the improvements in health from bioenergetic basics. One example of this is that of a couple who had tried unsuccessfully to achieve pregnancy. Upon scanning the husband, a BMP appeared in the energy areas of the ovaries and Fallopian tubes in his body, affecting his masculinity. They were depolarized and the wife became pregnant right away.

IMPORTANT CONTR INDICATIONS

In the event of a possible pregnancy, *do not place magnets in the vicinity of the ovaries and the uterus at the same time.*

If scanning people who have a pacemaker, Goiz tells them merely to place their hand over the pacemaker to protect it from magnetism. He scans them as usual.

Another example concerns **chemotherapy**. Goiz will treat almost every patient arriving at his clinic. But there is one group of patients he usually does not accept: those who have undergone chemotherapy. He says that the chemicals affect the cells so radically that bioenergetic basics is not effective. Other doctors—students of Goiz—have used magnets on former chemo patients. They do so mainly to provide palliative (soothing) treatment, not curative. At present, Goiz is working to devise a way to help these patients. Goiz does accept patients who have undergone radiation treatment if their immune system is still intact, which he decides on an individual basis by seeing if they respond to treatment.

FOLLOW-UP

Depending on the health of the person for whom bioenergetic basics is intended, another precaution can be advised. Since the body may be inundated with a plethora of dead micro organisms upon depolarization, their remains may give off toxins as they are expelled. The body is usually capable of getting rid of such toxic waste through normal processes of elimination and Goiz, as previously mentioned, generally does not even refer to a "healing crisis." Occasionally dead micro organisms and their toxins may be problematic.

It should be quite simple to avoid any adverse reactions. He may suggest a mild herbal laxative before going to bed that night. Other health practitioners suggest taking a tablespoon of Epsom salts in a glass of water the next morning. Parasites, fungi, and bacteria have lost their preferred magnetic environment and can no longer exist as before. If the bioenergetic basics session weakened but did not kill the micro organisms, they await the final blow from the body's own immune system. This, Goiz indicates, will usually happen within a week.

He sometimes recommends follow-up treatment for them:

<u>Parasites:</u> For parasites, he suggests that the patient take tablets or capsules of potassium for a few days to help the body finish killing the parasites that were weakened by bioenergetic basics

<u>Fungi:</u> Goiz prescribes systemic fungal remedies which are unavailable without a prescription. Depolarization greatly diminishes the amount of time they are taken. Other alternatives include herbal or homeopathic remedies after depolarization.

<u>Viruses:</u> As mentioned above, viruses may be eliminated very quickly. But they, as well as the other micro organisms, can leave toxins in their dying field, which the body will have to eliminate. To help the body detoxify these poisons, you can place a positive and a negative magnet over the thymus gland. The thymus is located under the clavicle above the beginning of the sternum--sort of where Tarzan bangs on his chest to show strength and valor. (This type of beating stimulates the thymus which plays a vital part in the immune system's response to sickness, and could be a fun, cathartic experience, especially if one does the jungle yodel while visualizing the body and helper cells whisking away the virus toxin "invaders" out of one's inner jungle!)

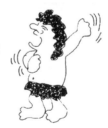

TARZAN BEATINGON CHEST TO STRENGTHEN THYMUS

55. Tarzan's thymus strengthener

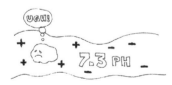

56. Bacterium struggling to survive in less alkaline, more balanced environment.

<u>Bacteria:</u> Being generally much larger than viruses and more robust in their makeup--having **bodies** rather than being merely particles with charges—they may need extra convincing that they are not wanted. With the negative magnet the body will have brought down the alkaline pH of their "living" and "breathing" medium to a level that they detest or that is toxic to them (like fish in polluted waters).

As with viruses, strengthening the thymus may help the body get rid of dead and dying bacteria. Since they sometimes do not die off as quickly as do viruses, Goiz might prescribe antibiotics. If you are not a medical doctor, there are natural or herbal remedies for stubborn bacteria that may be used in conjunction with magnets.

Over time, the indiscriminate use of antibiotics has caused some bacteria to develop highly resistant strains. Apparently, upon being impacted with magnets, the stability or resistant quality of the bacteria is destroyed. The bacteria become sensitive once again to antibiotic applications. The antibiotics (whether herbal or in drug form), therefore, are more effective, and smaller quantities are required.

In scanning, if you encounter a parasite linked with a biomagnetic pair, you know that there must be bacteria that the parasite was using as food. Look for bacteria, (which may also have been hidden or blocked from view by a more energetic parasite) then eliminate them so the parasite's food supply is cut off. You may add an herbal remedy or a small amount of medicine as the *coup de grace* for the parasite's passing. Remember that the amount of medicine or remedy may be less once the body is depolarized and better able to attack the pathogens.

GEOGRAPHY AND DEPOLARIZATION TIME

Goiz has found the closer to the equator we are, the less time it takes to obtain results from bioenergetic basics methods. At the equator, the time it takes for depolarization of a biomagnetic pair is very rapid--roughly two minutes. In Mexico City, the time needed is more than 12 minutes. Farther north, the magnets will have to be left on for longer time periods.

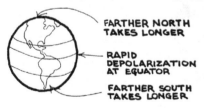

DEPOLARIZATION TIMES

FARTHER NORTH TAKES LONGER

RAPID DEPOLARIZATION AT EQUATOR

FARTHER SOUTH TAKES LONGER

57. Healing time and distance from equator

The necessary length of time can be determined by verifying when the biomagnetic pair has been depolarized and the legs are permanently the same length again. The author has found that, for example, in Utah at the northern latitude of 37° it takes about 20-25 minutes. In Brisbane, Australia, at a southern latitude of 27.5°, depolarization takes place about 12-15 minutes.

Goiz has also noted that certain areas at the same latitude have different depolarization rates, which may be due to the flow of electromagnetic energy around and in the earth, or, possibly to the quality of air, water, and sunshine. Magnetic cycles of sun spots are another potential influence on depolarization time. Investigative work could shed light on these phenomena.

The timing of when to remove the magnets has to be determined individually at each location. When in doubt, a good policy is to leave the magnets on longer. In Goiz' clinic in Mexico City, for example, he usually puts them on, goes to other patients, and then returns to remove them some 25-30 minutes later. That way the depolarization is assured without having to time them specifically.

FURTHER CLARIFICATIONS

When Goiz scans, he begins at the top of the head (as shown in the illustrations at front of book). He does the points around the skull, the face, and the neck, and goes down the body from there. Many of the biomagnetic pairs are bilaterals or doubles, *i.e.*, their identification is a repetition, such as Armpit/Armpit or Cheekbone/Cheekbone. Usually one of the points is on the right side of the body and the other on the left on the indicated organ or body part. If both points are located on a single organ or body part, that will be shown on the list (such as Bladder/Bladder or Spleen/Spleen).

Some areas of the body contain more than one pair. For example, the kidney--right or left--can hold tetanus (Kidney/Kidney), diabetes mellitus (Right Kidney/Duodenum), malaria (Cheekbone/Opposite Kidney), intestinal dysfunction (Kidney/Opposite Sacral), and three special pairs with one point at the kidney, Goiz, Machin, and Ale. If the person's leg shortens upon scanning the kidney, then you must check the various possible matching points one by one. In the case of a polarized kidney, you would need to scan both kidneys, the duodenum, the cheekbones, the sacral area, as well as special pairs Goiz (parietal), Machin (ureter), and Ale (renal capsule on same side), to know which kidney BMP is involved.

If one polarized point is discovered during scanning but none of the other possible partner points listed in the body catalog cause the leg length to change, don't despair! Check in the Index under the name of the first polarized point and you should find other possible combinations. (For instance, if the sacrum point is discovered upon scanning, but neither sacrum nor femur appear to be the other half of the BMP, checking the index will reveal that Kidney/Interiliac are also possible partner points.)

In the Body Catalog, most of the BMPs are listed with the point on the right side of the body *first*, but in some cases the point on the left side of the body may be first (depending on Goiz's discovery of it.) Also, if the situation arises that you have depolarized a BMP, and on rechecking later, the same pair appears, it may mean you incorrectly depolarized the first time and need to redo it.(Know that no harm has been done by incorrectly placing the magnets.) Retry and check the heels very carefully. If the same pair appears again, take a look at outside influences such as stress, diet, electromagnetic interference at the home or workplace, an infected pet or partner, a dirty toothbrush, etc., because the person might just be getting re-infected or traumatized by other elements.

Bioenergetic basics may seem complicated at first. It takes dedication and time to learn. But the benefits of improved health with the ease of discovery of existing imbalances that may lead to disease (without expensive lab work) make the efforts worthwhile, and the skill, once learned, can serve you throughout life. By doing one BMP at a time, you get much good information. With practice your accuracy improves in placing the magnets, your ability to check the lengths of the legs becomes automatic and it takes you less time to scan.

Do not be alarmed if it takes more than an hour or two when first beginning to scan. Knowledge of anatomy and physiology will grow as you keep scanning. Visual aids can help as well. See the appendix at the end of the book for more information, and also visit our website www.bioenergeticbasics.com. We are constantly working to make bioenergetic basics easier and more user friendly. As new pairs become known, they will be posted on the website for you.

> Bioenergetic basics may seem complicated at first. It takes dedication and time to learn. But the benefits of improved health at low cost, and the ease of discovery of existing diseases make the effort worthwhile.

CHAPTER 16
CONCLUSIONS

Through proper bioenergetic basics you can become an artist of energy who stimulates and creates well being for yourself, friends, and family. Such creation can be likened to a fine symphony or oil painting. With bioenergetic basics we have the chance to help the body create wonderful wellness.

Bioenergetic basics can reduce fear of illness and dependency on others and on chemicals and drugs. In one sense we learn how the body can change its own bioenergetic "melody" from that of a tragic opera to that of a peppy march or peaceful sonata that creates a tranquil environment where disturbing micro organisms feel uncomfortable and out of place. We can have greater control over our lives and our longevity when we manage our energy and our magnetism for wellness.

Restoring polarized areas of the body to energetic equilibrium may serve as the "stitch in time" saving us from not just nine, but over 250 chances for disease. Saving us, too, from unfruitful effort spent addressing only symptoms, as we often did before being illuminated by the concept of duality in bioenergy.

Bioenergetic basics offers economic power and freedom as well. Goiz gives us the way *he* diagnoses and treats disease conditions. His teachings may mean less money spent on medicines or expensive lab tests. The need for certain surgeries may be reduced or eliminated. Cancers and many syndromes may be alleviated. Such knowledge affords us the opportunity to experience a life of dynamic wellness that is exciting and worth living.

In writing this book, the author has desired to bring concepts new to the English-speaking world, specifically including these ideas of Isaac Goiz. Beginning with an introduction of how the biomagnetic pair was discovered, the author discussed briefly the importance of duality in magnetism and pH. A short history of magnets and a look at magnetism in the earth and in the body provided the platform to launch the discussion of the biomagnetic pairs. The details of the important topic of scanning followed with various references and examples to help the reader. With the author's organization of the list of "conditions and possible BMPs for depolarization," much time can be saved in trying to locate specific BMPs. The Body Catalog, also organized alphabetically, gives the reader an easy-to-use reference, something that was formerly lacking and greatly needed by students of bioenergetic basics.

The fact that you have this basic guidebook in your hands means that you are on the pathway for beautiful artistry of bioenergy in your inner space. Congratulations! And best wishes for Dynamic Wellness!

DISCLAIMER

The biomagnetic pair information contained in this section stems from the discovery and subsequent research of Isaac Goiz Duran. The author is not a licensed physician and offers this information for educational purposes only. The author disclaims any liability or loss in connection with this information. The biomagnetic pairs themselves, as well as the drawings of their approximate location in no way intend to replace or substitute actual licensed medical evaluation and/or treatment.

CHAPTER 17
ALPHABETIZED LIST OF CONDITIONS AND POSSIBLE BMPS FOR DEPOLARIZATION

ALWAYS SCAN FIRST!

ALPHABETICAL LIST OF CONDITIONS/ELEMENTS AND
suggested BIOMAGNETIC PAIRS FOR DEPOLARIZATION

*Prior Scanning Is **Essential** for Locating Goiz Biomagnetic Pairs*

ELEMENTS	BIOMAGNETIC POLARIZATIONS
Abdominal distention	Hepatic Ligament/Right Kidney (Adeno virus)
Abscessed lung tuberculosis	See Tuberculosis.
Abscesses	Supra Spinal/Supra Spinal (*Mycobacterium tuberculosis*); of sinus: Esophagus/Esophagus (Influenza virus) plus Mediastinum/Mediastinum (*Proteus mirabilis* bacteria) plus Costal/Liver (*Borrelia* bacteria)
Acid indigestión	See Gastric and Gastritis.
Acid urine (uric acid)	Right Kidney/Duodenum (Diabetes mellitus); Pancreas Tail/Kidney
Acne, common	Epiploon/Epiploon; also sexual organ dysfunctions
Actinomyces bacteria	Bursa/Bursa (found in women with IUD in place, for example)
Addison's disease	Adrenal/Adrenal

Adeno virus (hard to detect—likes to pair up with parvovirus)	Hepatic Ligament/Right Kidney.
Adenohypophysis acromegaly	Cranial/Cranial (Anthrax bacillus) plus Spleen/Liver (Common *Brucella* bacteria) plus Thymus/Parietal (Rubeola virus)
Adrenal problems	Adrenal/Adrenal; Pineal/Pineal (magnets horizontally) due to trauma to Pineal
Aerobacter aeruginosa bacteria	Antipole/Antipole
Aggression	Rachidian Bulb/Cerebellum (Newcastle virus); Right Temporal/Right Temporal (Many criminals have this.)
AIDS	Thymus/Rectum; Once depolarized, can do Index/Index to erase memory from blood cells—may take up to 7 months of effort.
AIDS, false	Eye/Eye (Cytomegalovirus); Eyelid/Eye (*Neisseria catarrallis* bacteria); Hepatic Ligament/Right Kidney (Adenovirus); See Thymus/Rectum and also HIV.
AIDS, false (1)--Daniel syndrome)	Mediastinum/Mediastinum (*Proteus mirabilis* bacteria) plus Pleura/Liver (Hepatitis B)
AIDS, false (2)	Carina/Carina (Aphthous virus) plus Cervical Plexus/Cervical Plexus (*Streptococcus fecalis*)
Alimentary canal bleeding, high, in adult	Stomach/Adrenals (Measles virus)
Allergies	Subclavian/Subclavian (Diphtheria bacillus); Pancreas/Stomach (special pair); Adrenal/Front of body
Alzheimer's	Calcaneus/Calcaneus (*Rickettsia* bacteria) plus Wrist/Wrist (*Rickettsia* bacteria)
Alzheimer's, false	Cheekbone/Kidney (*Plasmodium vivax*) plus Thymus/Parietal (Rubeola virus) plus Mastoid/Mastoid (*Filaria* worm parasite); Parietal/Parietal (Encephalitis virus); Pituitary/Bladder (Common dengue virus); Rachidian bulb/Bladder (Hemorrhagic dengue virus); Rachidian bulb/Cerebellum (Newcastle virus); Rachidian bulb/Thyroid (Meningitis virus); Temporal/Temporal (Typhus exanthematique virus); Armpit/Armpit (Rabies virus); Ulna/Ulna (Herpes 3)

Amenorrhea (suppression, absence of menstruation)	Pituitary/Ovary
Anasaki virus	Descending colon/Pancreas tail (from eating raw fish—gives stomach problems)
Anemia	Scan all points first; Sternum/Adrenals, to regulate number of red blood cells; ask from whence comes the bleeding and do a magnet there and one on kidney for a temporary pair
Anorexia	Esophagus/Esophagus (*Fasciolopsis buski* parasite); Perihepatic/Perihepatic (*Morganella typhus* bacteria)
Anthrax bacillus	Cranial/Cranial
Aphthous virus	Carina/Carina (milk products) often confused with Herpes 3 and 4
Arterial hypertension	Carotid/Carotid (Special pair); Jugular/Jugular (Not regular pair)
Arthritis	Mandible/Mandible (*Neisseria gonorrhea* bacteria)
Arthritis, deforming rheuma-toid	Dorsal/Lumbar (*Meningococcus* bacteria) plus Mandible/Mandible (*Gonococcus* bacteria)
Arthritis, Differential diagnosis	Middle Deltoid/Middle Deltoid (*Treponema palidum* bacteria)
	Scapula/Scapula (*Mycobacterium lepra*) plus Tonsil/Tonsil (Herpes 2 virus associated with chicken pox) plus Deltoid/Deltoid (*Treponema palidum* bacteria)
	Deltoid/Deltoid (*Treponema palidum* bacteria causing syphilis) plus Quadrate/Quadrate (*Treponema palidum* bacteria) plus Malar/Malar (*Gonococcus* bacteria) plus Urethra/Urethra (Corona virus); Calcaneus/Calcaneus or Wrist/Wrist (*Rickettsia* bacteria); Pancreas Head/Adrenals or Pericardium/Pericardium (*Staphylococcus aureus*); Infra Armpit/Infra Armpit or Pleura/Pleura-two sides (Viral pleuritis); Carina/Carina (Aphthous virus); Pudendal/Pudendal plus Parodtid/Parotid (Viral parotiditis); Pituitary/Bladder or Rachidian Bulb/Bladder (Dengue virus); Cheekbone/Opposite Kidney (Malaria); Occipital/Occipital (Epstein-Barr virus); Temporal/Temporal or Major Trochanter/Major Trochanter (Typhus virus); Cervical Plexus/Cervical Plexus (*Streptococcus fecalis*)

Aspergillus fungus	Canthus/Canthus
Asthma	See Goiz special pair; Adrenals/Front of Body
Asthma, false	Armpit/Armpit (Rabies virus); Subclavian/Subclavian (Diphtheria bacillus)
Astrocytoma (brain tumor of star-shaped cells)	Scapula/Scapula (*Mycobacterium lepra*) plus Colon,Descending/Colon, Descending (*Enterobacter cloacae*) plus Armpit/Armpit (Rabies virus) plus Parietal/Colon, Transverse (*Entomoeba histolytic* parasite)
Atherosclerosis	Countercaecum/Countercaecum (cholesterol); Esophagus/Esophagus plus Spleen/Spleen (triglycerides)
Auriculoventricular shunt persistence	Pericardium/Pericardium (*Staphylococcus aureus* bacteria) plus Cardia/Adrenal (*Streptococcus* B bacteria) plus Pancreas Head/Adrenal (*Staphylococcus aureus coag -*)
Bacteria	Aerobacter aeruginosa, *Actinomyces bacteria* *Bordatella pertussis (whooping cough)* *Borrelia* *Bovine tuberculosis* *Brucella* *Brucella abortus* *Chlamydia psittaci (pneumonia)* *Chlamydia trachomatis* *Clostridium malignum* *Clostridium perfringens* *Clostridium tetani* *Diphtheria bacillus* *Enterobacter cloacae* *Enterobacter pneumonia* *Enterococcus* *Escherichia coli* *Giardinella vaginalis* *Helicobacter pilori* *Klebsiella pneumonia* *Legionella* *Meningococcus bacteria*

	Morganella typhus
	Mycobacterium lepra
	Mycobacterium tuberculosis
	Neisseria gonorrhea
	Neisseralis catarrallis
	Neocardia americana
	Paratyphus bacillus
	Pasteurela
	Pneumococcus or pneumonia bacteria
	Proteus mirabilis
	Pseudomona aeruginosa
	Rickettsia
	Salmonella typhus
	Shigella
	Spirochete
	Spirochete E.
	Staphylococcus albus
	Staphylococcus aeruginosa
	Staphylococcus auerus coag +
	Staphylococcus aureus coag −
	Staphylococcus dorado coag +
	Staphylococcus epidermis
	Streptococcus A, B, C, fecalis, fragilis, G
	Syphilis bacteria
	Treponema palidum
	Trypanosoma cruzi
	Trypanosoma gambiense
	Tuberculosis
	Veillonella
	Vibrio cholera
	Whooping cough
	Yersinia pestis
	Yersinia pestis intestinal
	Yersinia pestis pneumonia
Balance	See Equilibrium.
Balantidium typhus parasite	Cervical 3/Supraspinal

Behavior changes	Occipital/Occipital (Epstein-Barr virus); Pancreas Body/Pancreas Tail (*Staphylococcus aureus cuag-*); see Special pair Goiz.
Belching	Stomach/Stomach
Belly, swollen	False pregnancy—see Roberta special pair
Best syndrome	Lachrymal/Lachrymal (Hemophylus influenza) plus Maxillary Sinus/Maxillary Sinus (Viral sinusitis) plus Eyelid/Eyelid (*Neisserria catarrallis* bacteria)
Bladder, problems	Pudendal/Pudendal (Parotiditis virus)
Bladder, Differential Diagnosis	Pudendal/Pudendal, etc. Bladder nerve similar to that of internal secretion glands, and its function can be altered by various micro-organism's toxins such as histamine, properdine, polypeptides, lysozime, urea, creatine, etc.
Blastocystis hominis fungus	Neck/Neck
Bleeding, coagulation	Hip/Hip (*Chlamydia pneumonia* bacteria)
Blindness	Parietal/Parietal (Encephalitis virus)
Blood cell, white, production and quality	Appendix/Thymus; Check in cases of leukemia.
Blood flow	Temple/Temple
Blood in urine	Ureter/Ureter (Varicella virus or chicken pox in adults); Urethra/Urethra (Corona virus); Kidney/Kidney (*Chlostridium tetani* bacteria)
Blood pressure, high	See Arterial hypertension, Cardiac problems, Hypertension, Circulation
Bloody discharge	Sternum/Liver
Bone disturbances	Parotid/Parotid (Lolita special pair)
Bordatella bacteria	Countercaecum/Countercaecum
Bordatella pertussis bacteria	Larynx/Larynx
Borrelia bacteria	Costal/Liver to Hepatic Duct (Hepatitis F--main factor in dysplasias)
Botulism	Pancreas Tail/Liver (*Clostridium botulinum* bacteria) (Can give Hepatitis H)
Bovine tuberculosis	Perirenal/Perirenal; is rare; in animals gives urinary symptoms (urinary insufficiency)

Brain, circulation disturbances	Temple/Temple
Brain, toxin	Wrist/Wrist (*Rickettsia* bacteria); Parietal/Parietal (Encephalitis virus); Rachidian Bulb/Thyroid (Meningitis) or Pineal/Rachidian Bulb (Guillan barre virus).
Breathing pathways disturbances	Adrenals/Rectum (*Leptospira* parasite)
Breathing problems	Polygon/Polygon (Reovirus); Adrenals/Front of body (Asthma); Colon, Ascending/Right Kidney (pneumonia); Caecum/Caecum (Haemophilus influenza); Caecum/Right Kidney (*Klebsiela pneumonia*); Chondral/Chondral (*Pneumosistis carini* fungus); Costal/Costal (*Proteus mirabilis*); Eyebrow/Eyebrow (Sincitial virus); Forehead Sinus/ Forehead Sinus (Viral sinusitis); Gallbladder/ Right Kidney (Common cold); Hiatus/Esophagus (*Enterobacter pneumonia* bacteria); Humerus/ Humerus (*Enterobacter pneumonia*); Larynx/Larynx (*Bordatella pertussis* bacteria); Mediastinum, inferior/ Mediastinum, superior (*Protus mirabilis* bacteria); Pituitary/Bladder (Common dengue virus); Pleura/ Pleura--1 side (*Pseudomona aeruginosa* bacteria); Pleura/Pleura--2 sides (Pleuritis virus); Popliteal/ Popliteal (*Pneumococcus* bacteria); Rachidian bulb/ Bladder (Hemorrhagic dengue virus); Spleen/ Spleen (*Yersinia pestis* bacteria); Spleen/Duodenum (Leukemia--often confused with brucellosis); Spleen/ Liver (*Brucellosis* bacteria); Subclavian/Subclavian (Diphtheria bacillus); Testicle/Testicle (*Yersinia pestis*); Trachea/Trachea (Influenza virus)
Breathing regulation	Cerebellum/Rachidian Bulb (Newcastle virus)
Bronchial problems	(Two types bronchial spasms-entrapped air or vascular supply: Parietal/Kidney (Goiz special pair); Temple/ Temple (Isaac special pair); Inferior Mediastinum/ Superior Mediastinum (*Proteus mirabilis*); Temple/ Temple; Carina/Carina;

Bronchial problems relating to air conditioners	Cervical Plexus/Cervical Plexus (*Streptococcus fecalis* bacteria)
Bronchiectasis (pulmonary)	(destruction of bronchial walls) Pleura/Pleura (Pleuritis virus) plus Colon, Ascending/Liver (*Klebsiella pneumonia* bacteria) plus Epiploon/Epiploon (*Streptococcus albus*)
Bronchitis	Scapula/Scapula (*Mycobacterium lepra*) infects 30% of Mexicans; Temple/Temple
Bronchitis with fever, similar to	Pleura/Pleura (Pleuritis virus) magnets on two sides
Bronchitis, chronic	Chondral/Chondral (*Pneumosistis carini* fungus)
Brucella abortus bacteria	Diaphragm/Kidney (This bacteria excites peritoneum and abortion occurs.)
Brucellosis or Maltese fever	Spleen/Liver
Brucellosis, confused with	Spleen/Duodenum (Leukemia)
Bruising	Sternum/Liver
Bulimia	Esophagus/Esophagus (*Fasciolopsis buski* parasite)
Bulimia connected with false pregnancy	Pole/Pole
Calcitonin (hormone made in the thyroid gland), production of	Parotid/Parotid (Lolita special pair)
Calcium absorption, ion production	Parotid/Parotid
Calcium intake regulation	Parathyroid/Parathyroid
Cancer, bone (osteosarcoma), inferior member	Scapula/Scapula (*Mycobacterium lepra*) plus Calcaneus/Calcaneus (*Rickettsia bacteria*) plus Sciatic/Sciatic (Polio virus) plus Tibia/Tibia (*Malassezia furfur*--aggressive fungus)
Cancer, bone (osteosarcoma), upper member	Scapula/Scapula (*Mycobacterium lepra*) plus Wrist/Wrist (*Rickettsia* bacteria) plus Ulna/Ulna (Herpes 3) plus Armpit/Armpit (Rabies virus)
Cancer, breast, left	Scapula/Scapula (*Mycobacterium lepra*) plus Pericardium/Pericardium (*Staphylococcus aureus* +) plus Armpit/Armpit (Rabies virus) plus Spleen/Liver (*Common Brucelllosis* bacteria)

Cancer, breast, right	Scapula/Scapula (*Mycobacterium lepra*) plus Appendix/Pleura (Staphylococcus aureus +) plus Pleura/Liver (Hepatitis B) plus Perihepatic/Perihepatic (Morganella typhus bacteria)
Cancer, cervical uterine	Scapula/Scapula (*Mycobacterium lepra*) plus Duodenum/Left Kidney (*Chlamydia trachomatis* fungus) plus Vagina/Vagina (Yersinia pestis bacteria) plus Rectum/Rectum (*Pseudomona aeruginosa* bacteria) plus Caecum/Caecum (*Trichomonas* parasite) plus Fallopian Tube/Fallopian Tube (Parvo virus); check also Hip/Hip (*Chlamydia pneumonia* bacteria) and *Pseudomona* or *yersinia,* which, if together, can give false cervical uterine cancer;
Cancer, false	Esophagus/Esophagus (*Fasciolopsis buski* parasite or Hepatic faciola which obstructs normal flow in liver)
Cancer, lung	*Scapula/Scapula (Mycobacterium lepra)* plus Poplitpeal/Popliteal (*Pneumococcus* bacterium) plus Supraspinal/Supraspinal (*Mycobacterium tuberculosis*) plus Carina/Carina (Aphthous virus)
Cancer, malignancy factor	Scapula/Scapula (*Mycobacterium lepra*)
Cancer, nerve cell, connective tissue	See Gliosarcoma.
Cancer, pancreas head	Scapula/Scapula (*Mycobacterium Lepra*) plus Pancreas Head/Adrenals (Staphylococcus aureus cuag -) plus Costodiaphragmatic/Costodiaphragmatic (*Trypanosoma cruzi* bacteria) plus Ureter/Ureter (Varicella virus)
Cancer, rectal	Scapula/Scapula (*Mycobacterium lepra*) plus Rectum/Rectum (*Pseudomona aeruginosa* bacteria) plus Colon, Ascending/Kidney (*Klebsiella pneumonia* bacteria) plus Prostate/Rectum (Papiloma virus)
Cancer, skin (melanoma)	Scapula/Scapula (*Mycobacterium lepra*) plus Colon, Descending/Colon, Descending (*Enterobacter clocae* bacteria) plus Carina/Carina (Aphthous virus) plus Brachial/Brachial (*Streptococcus* A) plus Bladder/Bladder (*Streptococcus* G)

Cancer, spinal chord	Scapula/Scapula (*Mycobacterium lepra*) plus Dorsal/Lumbar (*Pneumococcus* bacteria) plus Pleura/Pleura (Pleuritis virus) plus Diaphragm/Diaphragm (*Candida albicans* yeast-like fungus)
Cancer, testicle	Scapula/Scapula (*Mycobacterium lepra*) plus Testicle/Testicle (*Yersinia Pestis*) plus Prostate/Rectum (Papiloma virus) plus Colon, Descending/Colon, Descending (*Enterobacter cloacae* bacteria)
Cancer, uterus	Scapula/Scapula (*Mycobacterium lepra*) plus Vagina/Vagina (*Yersinia pestis* bacteria) plus Fallopian Tube/Fallopian Tube (Parvovirus) plus Countercaecum/Countercaecum (*Bordatella pertussis* bacteria)
Candida albicans fungus	Diaphragm/Diaphragm
Canker sores	Tongue/Tongue; Carina/Carina......
Cardiac insufficiency	Costodiaphragmatic/Costodiaphragmatic (Trypanosoma cruzi bacteria)
Cardiac problems	Pericardium/Pericardium (Staphylococcus aureus cuag+ bacteria) Esophagus/Esophagus (Fasciolopsis buski or Hepatic faciola)
Cardiomegaly (enlargement of the heart)	Pericardium/Pericardium (*Staphylococcus aureus*) plus Appendix/Pleura (*Staphylococcus aureus*) plus Cervical Plexux/Cervical Plexus (*Streptococcus fecalis*)
Cardiovascular problems, severe	Costodiaphragmatic/Costodiaphragmatic (*Trypanosoma cruzi* bacteria)
Carpal tunnel	Cervical/Dorsal (Special pair Pasciano)
Cataracts	Scapula/Scapula (*Mycobacterium lepra*) plus Malar/Malar (Enterovirus) plus Eye/Eye (Cytomegalovirus) or other virus; Parietal/Parietal (Encephalitis virus)
Catarrh	Kidney/Kidney (*Clostridium tetani* bacteria) Jugular/Jugular
Central nervous system	Pancreas Body/Pancreas Tail (*Staphylococcus aureus cuag-*)
Cerebral ataxia (lack of coordination)	Rachidian Bulb/Cerebellum (Newcastle virus)
Cerebral cysts	Parietal/Colon, Transverse (*Entomoeba histolytic* parasite)

Cerebral fever	Parietal/Parietal (Encephalitis virus)
Cerebral microcirculation	Temple/Temple
Cerebral problems	Pancreas/Pancreas (Special pair Ramses); Parietal/Opposite Kidney (Special pair Goiz)
Chagas disease, from fleas	Costodiaphragmatic/Costodiaphragmatic (*Trypanosoma cruzi* bacteria)
Chemotherapy	Violent to cells, causing biomagnetic and cellular disorganization; one year after chemo, can try Quadriceps/Quadriceps for alleviation
Chicken pox	Ureter/Ureter (Varicella virus); Ulna/Ulna (Herpes 3—associated with varicella virus, chicken pox)
Chills, recurring	Hand/Hand (*Plasmodium* parasite)
Chlamydia psittaci ("pneumonia") bacteria	The *Chlamydia* microorganisms live as parasites within the cell and have properties in common with both viruses and bacteria, and are classified as specialized bacteria) The psittaci illness is given by infected birds and sometimes called "parrot fever". Hip/Hip (Main cause of false cervical-uterine cancer if associated with *Pseudomona* or *Yersinia*)
Chlamydia trachomatis bacteria	Duodenum/Left Kidney
Cholesterol, high	Brachial/Brachial (*Streptococcus* A bacteria)
Cholic, hypogastric	Pylorus/Liver (Pin worm parasite) plus Trochanter, Minor/Trochanter, Minor (HIV 2) plus Chondral/Chondral (*Pneumocystis carini* fungus) plus Pancreas Head/Adrenals (*Staphylococcus aureus cuag* -)
Chronic diseases	Inguinal Nerve/Inguinal Nerve (HIV 3 virus reservoir—still under study)
Circulation, poor	Sternocleidomastoid/Sternocleidomastoid (Sympathetic nerve system dysfunction); also with constriction of blood vessels, can be Ureter/Ureter (Varicella virus)
Cirrhosis, liver	Perihepatic/Perihepatic (*Morganella typhus* bacteria), confused with cirrhosis in biopsies, as is on edge of liver; Ileosecal/Right Kidney (*Trichomonas* bacteria)
Clostridium botulinum bacteria	Pancreas Tail/Liver

Clostridium malignum	Supra Hepatic/Supra Hepatic
Clostridium perfringens bacteria	Stomach/Pylorus (bacteria, very aggressive)
Clostridium tetani bacteria	Kidney/Kidney; Jugular/Jugular
Cold virus, common	Gallbladder/Right Kidney (First check to make sure it is not an allergy.)
Cold sores	Commissure/Commissure
Colic	Kidney/Ureter (Special pair Machin); Pancreas Tail/Liver (*Chlostridium botulinum* bacteria)
Colitis	Right Pleura/Liver (Hepatitis B--curable); Sternocleidomastoid/Sternocleidomastoid; Duodenum/Duodenum
Colon, enlarged	Costal/Liver when combined with *Vibrio cholera*
Colon, irritable	Sternocleiomastoid/Sternocleidomastoid (Sympathetic dysfunction)
Conjunctiva, hemorrhagic	See Eye, Eyelid.
Conjunctivitis	Hepatic Ligament/Right Kidney (Adenovirus) plus Canthus/Canthus (Aspergillus fungus)
Constipation	Colon, Descending/Rectum (Special pair Olazo); Colon, Transverse/Bladder (*Vibrio cholera* bacteria); Iliac/Iliac (Special pair Elena)
Constriction of blood vessels, ureters	Ureter/Ureter (Varicella virus)
Convulsions, repeated	Ear/Ear (*Toxoplasma* gondii)
Convulsions, to stop	Pancreas/Pancreas (Special pair Ramses)
Corona virus	Urethra/Urethra
Cough	Lachrymal/Lachrymal (*Klebsiella pneumonia* bacteria)
Cough, chronic	Chondral/Chondral (*Pneumosistis carini* fungus); Larynx/Larynx (*Bordatella pertussis* bacteria); Subclavian/Subclavian (Diphtheria bacillus)
Cough, laryngeal-bronchitis-type	Spleen/Spleen (*Yersinia pestis* bacteria);Testicle/Testicle (*Yersinia pestis* bacteria); Vagina/Vagina (*Yersinia pestis* bacteria)
Coxsackievirus	Mango/Mango
Crisis, trauma	Adrenal/Adrenal; Kidney/Kidney

Cyst, pyronine	Ureter/Ureter (Varicella virus) plus Fallopian Tube/ Fallopian Tube (Parvo virus) plus Tibia/Tibia (*Malassezia furfur* aggressive fungus)
Cyst, right sinus	Suprahepatic/Suprhepatic (*Clostridium malignum* spore-forming bacteria needing no oxygen) plus Pleura/Liver (Hepatitis B virus)
Cystic fibrosis	A bacteria plus a virus; scan them out.
Cystic pulmonary fibrosis (allopathy declares "no known cure")	Popliteal/Popliteal (*Pneumococcus* bacteria) plus Dorsal/Lumbar (*Meningococcus* bacteria) plus Armpit/ Armpit (Rabies virus)
Cysticercosis	Sub diaphragm/Sub diaphragm, reservoir for; is Ecuador special pair. Cysticercus is pork tapeworm.
Cysticercus	Pork tapeworm from poorly cooked pork. See cysticercosis.
Cystitis	Ureter/Ureter (Varicella virus or chicken pox in adults); Ulna/Ulna (Herpes 3);
Cysts	Cranial/Cranial (*Anthrax* bacillus)
Cytomegalovirus	Eye/Eye
Deafness	Parietal/Opposite Kidney
Dehydration	Colon, Transverse/Bladder (*Vibrio cholera* bacteria)
Dengue, common	Pituitary/Bladder
Dengue, hemorrhagic	Rachidian Bulb/Bladder
Dental caries	Angle/Angle contributing factor
Dermatitis	Brachial/Brachial (*Streptococcus* A bacteria)
Diabetes	Quadriceps/Quadriceps (insecticide or bismuth intoxication, from)
Diabetes insipid	Pituitary/Rachidian Bulb--often good results
Diabetes mellitus	Trochanter, Major/Trochanter, Major (*Salmonella typhus* bacteria) Duodenum/Right Kidney (*Chlamydia trachomatis*)
Diabetes mellitus, juvenile	One needs to check all of the following: Dysfunction of growth hormone (Adrenals) and alterations of: Costal/Liver (*Borrelia* bacteria, usually from animals) plus Epiploon/Epiploon (*Staphylococcus albus*).

Diabetes, misdiagnosis of	Gallbladder Duct/Right Kidney (common cold virus) Hiatus/Right Testicle (*Helicobacter pilori* bacteria); Pancreas Head/Adrenals (*Staphylococcus aureus coag-*): Right Epiploon/Right Epiploon (*Streptococcus albus*) plus Left Epiploon/Left Epiploon (*Streptococcus albus*); from fleas: Costodiaphragmatic/Costodiaphragmatic (*Trypanozoma cruzi* bacteria) Trochanter, Major/ Trochanter, Major (*Salmonella typhus* bacteria); Duodenum/Left kidney (*Chlamydia trachomatis*); Hip/Hip (*Chlamydia pneumonia*); Caecum/Caecum (*Trichomonas*); Caecum/Caecum (Haemophilus influenza); Colon, Transverse/Bladder (*Vibrio cholera*); Parietal/Colon, Transverse (*Entamoeba histolytic* parasite); Pylorus/liver (*Enterobius vermicularis*-Pinworm); Achilles/Achilles (*Shigella* bacteria);Colon, Descending/ Liver (*Pasteurela* bacteria) Colon, Descending/Colon, Descending (*Enterobacter cloacae*); Costodiaphragmatic/ Costodiaphragmatic (*Trypanosoma cruzi*); Flank/Flank, Spleen/Spleen, Testicle/Testicle, Vagina/Vagina (all of which are *Yersinia pestis*)
Diaphragm disorders	Costal/Costal (Proteus mirabilis); Dorsal/Lumbar (*Meningococcus bacteria); Adrenal/Rectum (Leptospira parasite); Cardia/Adrenal (Streptococcus* B); Diaphragm/ Kidney (*Brucella abortus* bacteria); Esophagus/Esophagus (*Fasciolopsis buski* parasite); Kidney/Kidney (*Clostridium tetani* bacteria); Pancreas head/Adrenal (*Staphylococcus aureus coag-*); Bladder/Bladder (*Streptococcus* G bacterium); Stomach/Adrenals (Measles virus)
Diaphragm, paralysis of	Pineal/Rachidian Bulb (Guillan barre virus)
Diaphragmatic hernia	Hiatus/Right Testicle (*Helicobacter pilori* bacteria)
Diarrhea	Achilles Tendon/Achilles Tendon (*Shigella* parasite); Countercaecum/Countercaecum (*Bordatella* bacteria); Trochanter, Major/Trochanter, Major (*Salmonella typhus* bacteria); Malar/Malar (Enterovirus); Perihepatic/Perihepatic (*Morganella typhus* bacteria); Subclavian/Subclavian (Diphtheria bacillus); Colon, Transverse/Bladder (*Vibrio cholera* bacteria)

Digestion disturbances	Countercaecum/Countercaecum (*Bordatella* bacteria); Colon, Descending/Colon, Descending (*Enterobacter cloacae* bacteria); Esophagus/Esophagus (*Fasciolopsis buski* or hepatic faciola); Gallbladder Duct/Right Kidney (*Spirochete* bacteria); Hiatus/Right Testicle (*Helicobacter pilori* bacteria); Iliac/Iliac Special Pair; Lumbar Plexus/Lumbar Plexus; Trochanter, Major/Trochanter, Major (*Salmonella typhus* bacteria); Trochanter, Major/Kidney; Pancreas/Pancreas; Parotid/Parotid (See Lolita special pair); Polygon/Polygon (Reovirus); Stomach/Pylorus (*Clostridium perfringens* bacteria); Stomach/Stomach
Digestive problems, acute	Hand/Hand (*Plasmodium* parasite); Perihepatic/Perihepatic (*Morganella typhus* bacteria); Diaphragm Hole/Diaphragm Hole (middle area of diaphragm–*Giardia lamblia*)
Digestive system intoxication	Pancreas/Pancreas; (See Ramses special pair)
Digestive tract mucus	Adrenals/Rectum
Diphtheria bacillus	Subclavian/Subclavian
Distemper in puppies	Parietal/Parietal (Encephalitis virus)
Dizziness	Malar/Malar (Enterovirus); Mastoid/Mastoid (*Filaria* parasite); Ear, Middle/Ear, Middle (*Toxoplasma gondii*); Occipital/Occipital (Epstein-Barr virus); Pineal/Rachidian Bulb (Guillan barre virus--very contagious); Pole/Pole (Special pair); Rachidian Bulb/Cerebellum (Newcastle virus);
Duodenal dysfunction	Duodenum/Duodenum
Dwarfism, under-active growth process	Supraciliar/Rachidian Bulb (Special pair)
Dyslexia	Pole/Pole may be involved
Dysmenorrha (difficult or painful menstruation)	Pituitary/Ovary (Special pair)
Ear problems, chronic	Armpit/Armpit (Rabies virus) Also see Ramsay-Hunt syndrome.
Edema	Jugular/Jugular; Kidney/Kidney (*Clostridium tetani* bacteria)

Edema, general, main cause of	Subclavian/Subclavian (Diphtheria bacillus)
Epstein-Barr virus	Occipital/Occipital
Elbow pain	Cervical/Dorsal
Elbow, tennis	See Tennis elbow
Elephantitis	Ischium/Ischium (*Oncocercosis* parasite)
Emphysema	Scapula/Scapula (*Mycobacterium lepra*) plus Temple/ Temple (vascular dysfunction) (See special pair Isaac)
Encephalitis virus	Parietal/Parietal
Endometriosis	Uterus/Uterus (Special pair Roberta)
Energy problems,	Prostate/Rectum (If is in female, check her for energy problems in prostate and testicles area and if Prostate/Rectum is in male, check him for energy problems in area of ovaries, Fallopian tube, uterus as these energies are present and can cause problems)
Entamoeba histolytic parasite	Parietal/Colon, Transverse
Enterobacter cloacae (from mucous from dogs, cats, farm animals)	Colon, Descending/Colon, Descending
Enterobacter pneumonia	Humerus/Humerus
Enterobius vermicularis	See pin worm
Enterococcus bacteria	Lumbar plexus/Lumbar plexus
Enterovirus	Malar/Sternum; Malar/Malar (confused with HIV)
Epilepsy	Mastoid/Mastoid (*Filaria* parasite)
Epiploon	*Staphylococcus albus* (acne)
Epistaxis (nosebleed)	Caecum/Caecum (*Trichomonas* parasite); Cranial/ Cranial (*Anthrax*); Eye/Eye (Cytomegalovirus); Hip/ Hip (*Chlamydia pneumonia* bacteria) Lachrymal/ Lachrymal (*Klebsiella pneumonia* bacteria); Rachidian Bulb/Bladder (Hemorrhagic Dengue);
Epithelium, ulcers in	Tibia/Tibia (*Pityrosporum* or *versicolor* or *Malassezia furfur* fungus)
Equilibrium	Cerebellum/Rachidian Bulb (Newcastle virus) Malar/ Malar (Enterovirus); Mastoid/Mastoid (*Filaria* parasite); Middle Ear/Middle Ear (*Toxoplasmosis* parasite); Occipital/ Occipital (Epstein-Barr virus); Pineal/Rachidian Bulb (Guillan barre virus--very contagious); Pole/Pole (Special pair); Rachidian Bulb/Cerebellum (Newcastle virus)

Equilibrium, horizontal	Ear/Ear (*Toxoplasmosis* parasite)
Equilibrium, vertical	Pole/Pole (Special pair)
Erectile dysfunction	Penis/Penis; Thymus/Penis
Eruptions, flat, on chest, back, arms	Inguinal Nerve/Liver (Roseola virus)
Escherichia coli bacteria	Index Finger/Index Finger; Thymus/Liver (giving Hepatitis L)
Esophagus varicosities	Cardia/Adrenal (*Streptococcus* B)
Evan syndrome	Pylorus/Liver (Pin worm parasite) plus Duodenum/Left Kidney (*Chlamydia trachomatis* bacteria) plus Fallopian Tube/Fallopian Tube (Parvo virus) plus Trochanter/Trochanter (*Salmonella typhus*)
Exanthematis typhus virus	See typhus
Eye dysfunctions	Elbow/Elbow (Special pair Castaneda); Canthus/Canthus (*Aspergillus* fungus)
Eye hemorrhaging	Thymus/Parietal (Rubeola virus)
Eye lesions	Duodenum/Left Kidney (*Chlamydia trachomatis* fungus)
Eye tumors	Ischium/Ischium (*Oncocercosis* parasite)
Eye, corpulency in front of eye (Pterigones)	Malar/Sternum (Enterovirus); Mandible/Mandible (*Neisseria gonorrhea* bacteria); Middle Deltoid/Middle Deltoid (Syphilis); Duodenum/Left Kidney (*Chlamydia trachomatis* fungus); Quadrate/Quadrate (*Syphilis* bacillus)
Eyeball, eyelid bleeding (Hemorrhagic conjunctiva)	Sternum/Liver
Eyes, bulging (exophthalmos)	Thyroid/Thyroid
Eyes, varicose ulcers	Scapula/Scapula (*Mycobacterium lepra*)
Facial paralysis	Mandible/Mandible (*Neisseria gonorrhea* bacteria)
Faciola, hepatic	Esophagus/Esophagus (*Fasciolopsis buskii* parasite)
Fasciolopsis buski parasite	Esophagus/Esophagus
Fatigue	Adrenal/Adrenal; Occipital/Occipital (Epstein-Barr virus); Pineal/Rachidian Bulb (Guillan barre virus); Right Pleura/Liver (Hepatitis B, curable with magnets);

Fertility, female	Adductor/Adductor; Colon, Descending/Colon Descending Duodenum/Left Kidney; Dorsal 2/ Dorsal 2; Fallopian Tube/Fallopian Tube; Hip/ Hip; Kidney/Ureter; Ovary/Ovary; Ovary/Uterus; Popliteal/Popliteal; Pituitary/Ovary; Sacrum/Sacrum; Supra Pubic/Supra Pubic; Vagina/Vagina; Tensor/ Tensor; Check women and men for Papiloma virus. Both types of dengue can negatively affect ovaries and uterus. Renal capsule/Renal capsule can cause infertility if it blocksthe uterus.
Fertility, male	Parotid/Parotid; Pudendal/Pudendal; Penis/Thymus; Prostate/Prostate; Prostate/Rectum; Sacrum/Sacrum; Spleen/Spleen; Supra Pubic/Supra Pubic; Tensor, Tensor Testicle/Testicle; Ureter/Ureter
Fever	Exercise, anxiety, dehydration, anemia, infections, etc. may cause fever. Some possible pairs: Hepatic Ligament/Right Kidney (Adeno virus); Jugular/ Jugular; Kidney/Kidney (*Clostridium tetani* bacteria; Perihepatic/Perihepatic (*Morganella typhus* bacteria); Temporal/Temporal (Typhus exanthematique virus); Hand/Hand (*Plasmodium* parasite)
Fibromyalgia	Ureter/Ureter (Varicella virus) plus Cheekbone/ Kidney (*Plasmodium vivax protozoa* parasite); Kidney/ Pomulus; Cheekbone/Opposite Kidney (*Malaria protozoan* parasite)
Fibrosis, pulmonary	Dorsal/Lumbar (*Meningococcus* bacteria) plus Scapula/ Scapula (*Mycobacterium lepra*) plus Carina/Carina (Aphthous virus)
Filaria parasite	Mastoid/Mastoid
Fingers, fat or inflamed	Scapula/Scapula (*Mycobacterium lepra*)
Flatulence	Achilles Tendon/Achilles Tendon (*Shigella* parasite); Adrenals/Rectum (*Leptospira* parasite) Colon, Descending/Colon, Descending (*Enterobacter cloacae*); Kidney/Opposite Sacral (Intestinal dysfunction); Pancreas Tail/Liver (*Clostridium botulinum* bacteria)

Flush (sudden reddening of facial and neck skin)	Pylorus/Opposite Kidney
Foot fungus	Cava/Cava (*Trycophyte* fungus)
Frigidity, sexual	Atlas/Atlas (Special pair
Fungi	*Aspergillus* *Blastocystis hominis* *Candida albicans* *Cryptococcus* (in Prepineal/Bladder) *Foot* (*Trycophyte*) *Intestinal mycelia* *Malassezia furfur* (brown spots on skin) *Mycosporum* *Nail* (*Onchomycosis*) *Pityrosporum* *Pneumocystis carini* *Trycophyte* *Yeast*
Fungus, to rid body of	Index Finger/Index Finger (*Escherichia coli*) --put finger tip in center of magnet; Neck/Femur; Scan for each individual fungus separately.
Gait, uneven and staggering	Cerebellum/Rachidian Bulb (Newcastle virus)
Gall bladder problems	Supraspinal/Supraspinal (*Mycobacterium tuberculosis*)
Gall bladder stones	Scapula/Scapula (*Mycobacterium lepra*) plus Gall bladder/Gall bladder (viral reservoir)
Gangrene	Tibia/Tibia (*Pityrosporum versicolor* or *Malassezia furfur* fungus)
Gangrene, dry (problem of diabetes mellitus)	Scapula/Scapula (*Mycobacterium lepra*) plus Brachial/Brachial (*Streptococcus* A) or Bladder/Bladder (*Streptococcus* G) plus Urethra/Urethra (Corona virus)
Gangrene, moist	Scapula/Scapula (*Mycobacterium lepra*) plus Kidney/Kidney (*Clostridium tetani* bacteria) plus Tibia/Tibia (*Malassezia furfur*--an aggressive fungus)
Gas, intestinal	See flatulence
Gastric insufficiency	Costodiaphragmatic/Costodiaphragmatic (*Trypanosoma cruzi* bacteria)

Gastric reflux, main cause	Pancreas Head/Adrenals (*Staphylococcus aureus coag-*)
Gastritis, main cause of	Adrenals/Stomach (measles virus) together with Helicobacter pilori
Gastritis, severe, followed by gastric ulcers	Hiatus/Right Testicle (*Helicobacter pilori* bacteria)
Gastroenteritis, chronic (Leny syndrome)	Fallopian Tube (Parvo virus) plus Urethra/Urethra (Corona virus) plus Colon, Ascending/Left Kidney (*Klebsiela pneumonia* bacteria) plus Cervical 3/ Supraspinal (*Balantidium typhus* parasite)
Giardia lamblia	Diaphragm hole/Diaphragm hole (middle area of diaphragm) giving severe digestive problems
Giardinella vaginalis bacteria	Tensor/Tensor
Gingivitis	Eyelid/Eyelid (*Neisseria catarrallis* bacteria); Mandible/Mandible (*Neisseria gonorrhea* bacteria)
Glandular disorders	Cervical/Sacrum; Scan points on and around specific glands.
Glaucoma	Lachrymal/Lachrymal (Klebsiella pneumonia bacteria) plus Malar/Malar (Enterovirus) plus Canthus/Canthus (*Aspergillus* fungus)
Gliosarcoma (glioblastoma)— cancer of connective tissue of nerve cells	Scapula/Scapula (*Mycobacterium lepra*) plus Colon, Descending/Colon, Descending (*Enterobacter cloacae*) plus Thymus/Parietal (Rubeola virus) plus Fallopian Tube/Fallopian Tube (Parvo virus) plus Caecum/ Caecum (*Tricomonas*)
Goiter	Thyroid/Thyroid
Gonorrhea	Mandible/Mandible (*Neisseria gonorrhea* bacteria)
Groin, itching	Achilles Tendon/Achilles Tendon (*Shigella* parasite)
Growth process, underactivity	Supraciliar/Rachidian Bulb (Special pair)
Guillan barre virus	Pineal/Rachidian Bulb; Wrist/Wrist
Hair falling out (alopecia areata)	Tongue/Tongue (Mange or scabies) See also Psoriasis.
Hair, excess of body or facial in women	Testicle/Testicle (*Yersinia pestis* bacteria)
Halitosis	Pancreas Head/Adrenals (*Staphylococcus aureus coag-*)

Hands, trembling	Thyroid/Thyroid
Hanta virus	Mole/Kidney of same side--Check moles over entire body.
Headache	Achilles/Achilles (*Shigella* parasite); Cerebellum/Rachidian Bulb (Newcastle virus); Colon, Transverse/Bladder (*Vibrio cholera* bacteria); Malar/Malar (Enterovirus); Temple/Temple (hypertension-cerebral circulation); Temporal/Temporal (*Typhus exanthematique*); Temporal, Left/Colon, Transverse (Structural dysfunction); Thymus/Parietal (Rubella virus); Thyroid/Rachidian Bulb (Meningitis virus)
Headache, chronic, main cause of	Temporal/Temporal (*Typhus exanthematique* virus)
Headache, in women	Cervical/Sacrum; from sex, Sternocleidomastoid/Sternocleidomastoid, as sexual organs irritate parasympathetic nerves, causing headache. Also Colon, Descending/Colon, Descending; Ureter/Ureter (Varicella virus or chicken pox in adult women. The autonomic nervous system, sympathetic and parasympathetic nervous systems run along the length of the spine up to the neck or head. With this or other virus or bacteria in same area, pain runs up spine, causing headache.
Headache, migraine	Temple/Temple plus Scapula/Scapula (*Mycobacterium lepra*)
Hearing, to improve	Ear, Upper/Ear, Upper
Heart arrhythmia	Costodiaphragmatic/Costodiaphragmatic (*Trypanosoma cruzi* bacteria); Pericardium/Pericardium (*Staphylococcus aureus coag+* bacteria)
Heart attacks, provoked by *Streptococcus* A bacteria	Coronaria/Left Lung
Heartburn	Can be reflux: Pancreas Head/Adrenals (*Staphylococcus aureus coag-*)
Heart disorder, from fleas	Costodiaphragmatic/Costodiaphragmatic (*Trypanosoma cruzi* bacteria)

Heart taquicardia (excessive velocity)	Sinoatrial-ventricular node of heart/Left Kidney
Helicobacter pilori bacteria	Hiatus/Right Testicle
Haemophilus influenza	Caecum/Caecum
Hemorrhoids	In women, Colon, Descending/Colon, Descending (*Enterobacter cloacae*)
Hepatic abscess	Parietal/Colon, Transverse (*Entamoeba histolytic* parasite) plus Perihepatic/Perihepatic (Morganella typhus)
Hepatic amoeba parasite	Liver/Left Kidney (*Hepatic amoeba* parasite--caused when amoeba go from pylorus to liver)
Hepatic cirrhosis	Right Kidney/Liver (*Morganella typhus*). Find out what % of organ is destroyed. Liver can regenerate.
Hepatic Syndrome	Spleen/Liver (Common brucellosis bacteria) plus Colon, Descending/Liver (*Pasteurela* bacteria-giving Hepatitis A) plus Liver/Liver (Hepatitis C)
Hepatitis A (Liver is + in all hepatitis/—check also Pancreas Tail/Liver (Botulism) and Spleen/Liver (Brucella) with all hepatitis.	Colon, Descending/Liver (*Pasteurela* bacteria) (Liver virus RNA type, is positive point)
Hepatitis B (See above under Hepatitis A)	Right Pleura/Liver--(DNA virus) If Right Pleura/Liver is detected, must also depolarize Prada special pair (reservoir), Gall bladder/Gall bladder
Hepatitis C (See above under Hepatitis A)	Liver/Liver (from toxins)
Hepatitis D (See above under Hepatitis A)	Duodenum/Liver (Specialized bacteria *Chlamydia trachomatis*, which lives in membrane lining eye and lining of urine passage or urethra and lower end of uterus, causing conjunctiva to swell, gives venereal disease, is sexually transmitted, can cause sterility)
Hepatitis E (See above under Hepatitis A)	Colon, Ascending/Liver (*Klebsiela* bacteria)
Hepatitis F (See above under Hepatitis A)	Costal/Liver (Borrelia)

Hepatitis G (See above under Hepatitis A)	Colon, Transverse/Liver (*Vibrio cholera* bacteria)
Hepatitis H (See above under Hepatitis A)	Pancreas Tail/Liver (Botulism)
Hepatitis I (See above under Hepatitis A)	Spleen/Liver (*Brucella*)
Hepatitis J (See above under Hepatitis A)	Pylorus/Liver (Pin worm)
Hepatitis K (See above under Hepatitis A)	Pancreas Head/Liver (*Staphylococcus aureus* -)
Hepatitis L (See above under Hepatitis A)	Thymus/Liver (*E. coli* bacteria)
Hernia, hiatus	Cardia/Mastoid plus Mediastinum/Mediastinum
Herpes 1 virus, associated with chicken pox	Colon, Ascending/Colon, Descending
Herpes 2 virus, associated with chicken pox	Tonsil/Tonsil
Herpes 3	Ulna/Ulna
Herpes 4	Calyx/Ureter
Herpes 5 virus	Commissure/Commissure
Herpes 6, viral infection	Inguinal Nerve/Liver (Roseola virus); Femoral Nerve/Femoral Nerve
Herpes 7	Chiasm/Chiasm
Herpes 8	Chin/Chin
Hiatal hernia	Hiatus/Right Testicle (*Helicobacter* pilori)
Hip or femur head degeneration	Countercaecum/Countercaecum (Bordatella bacteria)
Histoplasma capsulatum fungus	Esophagus/Left side of Bladder
HIV 1	If Thymus/Rectum is detected, depolarize also Prada special pair (reservoir), Gall Bladder/Gall Bladder, and Ale special pair (reservoir), Kidney/Renal Capsule.

HIV 2	Adductor/Adductor—not true AIDS as it does not affect thymus; gives vaginal and urethral disorders in women
HIV 3 virus	Inguinal Nerve/Inguinal Nerve (still under study) If found, also depolarize Gall Bladder/Gall Bladder (reservoir) and Kidney/Renal Capsule (Reservoir, special pair)
HIV 3, HIV 4	Trochanter, Lesser/ Trocanter, Lesser If found, also depolarize Gall Bladder/Gall Bladder and Kidney/ Renal Capsule (reservoirs).
HIV Reservoir	Gall Bladder/Gall Bladder (Prada special pair and Kidney/Renal Capsule (Ale special pair)
Hodgkin's disease (cancer of neck), main cause of	Subclavian/Subclavian (Diphtheria bacillus)
Hodgkin's disease (lymphore-ticuloma)	Scapula/Scapula (*Mycobacterium leprae*) plus Subclavian/Subclavian (Diphtheria bacillus) plus Carina/Carina (Aphthous virus) plus Dorsal 2/ Dorsal2 (*Legionella* bacteria)
Hodgkin's, false (1)	Tongue/Tongue (Mange or scabies) plus Esophagus/ Esophagus (Influenza virus) plus Quadrate/Quadrate (*Treponema palidum* bacteria) plus Armpit/Armpit (Rabies virus)
Hodgkin's, false (2)	Subclavian/Subclavian (Diphtheria bacillus) plus Larynx /Larynx (*Bordatella pertussis* bacillus) plus Colon, Ascending/Liver (*Klebsiela pneumonia* bacteria) plus Carina/Carina (Aphthous virus)
Hookworm parasite	Gallbladder Duct/Right Kidney
Hormonal dysfunction	Thymus/Adrenal (Echeverria special pair) If this is present, check to see which are the hormones affected.
Hormone production	Parotid/Parotid (Special pair Lolita) If found, check also for Pudendal/Pudendal, which can cause infertility in males.
Hot flashes	Pylorus/Opposite Kidney
HTLV virus	Supra Pubic/Supra Pubic

Huntington's chorea (a supposed "inherited" abnormality leading to insanity)	Thymus/Parietal (Rubeola virus) plus Rachidian Bulb/ Cerebellum (Newcastle virus) plus Occipital/ Occipital (Epstein-Barr virus) plus Parietal/Parietal (Encephalitis virus)
Hypertension	Jugular/Jugular (*Clostridium tetani* bacteria); Temple/Temple (special pair); Costodiaphragmatic/ Costodiaphragmatic (*Trypanosoma cruzi* parasite)
Hypertension due to organ blockage	Costodiaphragmatic/Costodiaphragmatic (Trepanosoma cruzi)
Hypocalcemia (deficiency of calcium ions)	Parathyroid/Parathyroid Also see Goiz special pair.
Hypokalemia	Pancreas Tail/Liver (*Clostridium botulinum* bacteria) plus Pancreas Head/Adrenal (*Staphylococcus aureus coag* -)
Hypophyseal adenoma	Cranial/Cranial (*Anthrax* bacillus) plus Malar/Malar (*Enterovirus*) plus Eye/Eye (Cytomegalo virus) plus Eyelid/Eyelid (*Neisseria catarrallis* bacteria)
Hyporexia (chronic low appetite)	Esophagus/Esophagus (*Fasciolopsis buski* parasite)
Immune deficiency	Appendix/Thymus, special pair; Canthus/Canthus (Aspergillus fungus)
Immune difficiency, main cause	Mediastinum, Inferior/Mediastinum, Superior (*Proteus mirabilis*)
Immune system, to heighten	Index Finger/Index Finger (*Escherichia coli*)
Implantation in pregnancy	Uterus/Ovary (Duran special pair)
Incontinence	Rachidian Bulb/Bladder (Dengue virus, hemorrhagic); Bladder/Bladder (*Streptococcus* G bacteria)
Infections, prone to	Adrenal/Adrenal Also positive and negative on thymus.
Infertility, main cause of in females	Fallopian Tube/Fallopian Tube (Parvovirus); Also see Fertility.
Inflammation symptoms from navel down to heel	Calcaneus/Calcaneus (*Rickettsia* bacteria)
Inflammation symptoms, from navel up to head	Wrist/Wrist (*Rickettsia* bacteria)

Influenza virus	Trachea/Trachea
Ingrid syndrome	Renal Capsule/Renal Capsule (*Proteus mirabilis* bacteria) plus Ureter/Ureter (Varicella virus) plus Neck/Neck (*Blastocystis hominis* fungus)
Injury, blow or wound	Negative at site of injury, positive on kidney of same side for 30 minutes. Then if pain continues, maintain negative at injury site for pain reduction.
Insect bites, stings including scorpion	Kidney/Kidney
Insecticide toxins	Quadriceps/Quadriceps (Special pair Magda)
Insomnia	Armpit/Armpit (Rabies virus); Parietal/Colon, Transverse (*Entomoeba histolytic* parasite); Rachidian Bulb/Rachidian Bulb
Insulin	Parotid/Parotid
Intestinal parasites	Gallbladder Duct/Right Kidney (*Spirochete* bacteria); Take potassium after depolarizing.
Intestinal amoebeasis parasite with vomit or metal taste in mouth	Pylorus/Left Kidney
Intestinal infection	Hepatic ligament/Right Kidney (Adenovirus)
Intestinal mycelia fungus	Pylorus/Ureter
Intestinal obstruction	Colon, Ascending/Liver (*Klebsiella pneumonia* bacteria) plus Colon, Transverse/Liver (Hepatitis G) plus Iliac/Iliac (Intestinal dysfunction); Colon, Descending/Rectum (special pair)
Intestinal problems	Pancreas Tail/Liver (*Clostridium botulinum* bacteria); Thymus/Rectum (*E. coli*); Kidney/Sacrum (intestinal dysfunction); Ileocecal Valve /Right Kidney (*Trichomonas* bacteria); Hiatus/ Right Testicle (*Helicobacter pilori* bacteria); Pituitary/ Rachidian Bulb (Diabetes insipid); Duodenum/Duodenum (glandular dysfunction); Adrenal/Rectum (*Leptospira* parasite); Pancreas Tail/Liver (Botulism); Colon, Transverse / Bladder (*Vibrio cholera* bacteria); Stomach/Stomach (Dysfunction);

	Colon, Descending/Colon, Descending (*Enterobacter cloacae*); Ulna/Ulna (Herpes 3); Trochanter, Major/ Trochanter, Major (*Salmonella typhus* bacteria); Countercaecum/ Countercaecum (*Bordatella pertussis* bacteria); Ileocecal Valve/Ileocecal Valve (Special pair); Malar/Malar (Enterovirus); Stomach/Adrenals (Measles virus--main cause of gastritis); Subclavian/ Subclavian (Diphtheria bacillus); Perihepatic/ Perihepaic (Morganela typhus); Esophagus/ Esophagus (*Fasciolopsis buski* parasite); Colon, Transverse/Liver (Hepatitis G); Sternocleidomastoid/Sternocleidomastoid (Dysfunction); Colon, Descending/Liver (Hepatitis A)
Intestinal virus	Mango/Mango (Coxsackievirus)
Intoxication	Ear, Upper/Ear, Upper (Special pair Leni)
Intoxication, bismuth insecticides, poisons	Quadriceps/Quadriceps
Intoxication, medication	Pylorus/Pylorus
Intracranial tumors	Mastoid/Mastoid (*Filaria* parasite)
Irritability	Occipital/Occipital (Epstein-Barr virus); Temporal/ Temporal (Typhus exanthematique virus)
Joint pain (for all joints)	Cheekbone/Opposite Kidney (*Malaria protozoan* parasite) In all joints, check for syphilis.
Joint problems, non infectious	Right Inguinal Nerve (+ pole)/Joints (- pole); Sacrum/Sacrum (*Proteus mirabilis* bacteria)
Joint, swelling from physical trauma	Joint/Kidney of same side
Kaposi sarcoma	Mediastinum/Mediastinum (*Proteus mirabilis* bacteria) plus Pleura/Liver (Hepatitis B virus) plus Urethra/ Urethra (Corona virus)
Keloids	See scars.
Keratoconus (conelike bulge on cornea)	Supraspinal/Supraspinal (*Mycobacterium tuberculosis*) plus Cheekbone/Kidney (*Plasmodium vivax* parasite) plus Armpit/Armpit (Rabies virus)

Kidney infection	Kidney -/Parietal +
Kidney problems, differential diagnosis	Canthus/Canthus (Aspergillus fungus); Kidney-/Parietal+; Supra Spinal/Supra Spinal (*Mycobacterium tuberculosis*) often fatal, can be relieved with this pair
Kidney stones, cause	See renal lithiasis. Scapula/Scapula (Mycobacterium lepra) Magnets may not break them up as the deposit is inert, won't react to the magnetic energy.
Kidney stones, passing	Kidney/Ureter to ease pain (Special pair Machin)
Klebsiella bacteria	Colon, Ascending/Liver (Hepatitis E)
Klebsiella pneumonia bacteria	Caecum/Right Kidney; Colon, Ascending/Right Kidney; Lachrymal/Lachrymal
Laryngeal problems	Mediastinum, Inferior/Mediastinum, Superior (*Proteus mirabilis*)
Laryngitis	Lachrymal/Lachrymal (Klebsiella pneumonia bacteria)
Larynx cancer, false	Tongue/Tongue (Mange or scabies)
Larynx problems	Appendix/Pleura of same side (Staphylococcus aureus coag+bacteria)
Legionella bacteria	Dorsal2/Dorsal 2
Leishmania parasite	Deltoid/Kidney of same side
Leprosy	Scapula/Scapula (*Mycobacterium lepra*)
Leptospira parasite	Adrenals/Rectum
Lethargy, sleepiness	Pancreas/Pancreas (Special pair)
Leukemia	Spleen/Duodenum (confused with Brucellosis at times, Spleen/Liver) In addition to Spleen / Duodenum, check for Appendix/Thymus, involved with white blood cell (Angeles special pair)
Libido alterations	Atlas/Atlas (Rigidity or sexual overstimulation—special pair)
Lipoma	Associated with Parotid. Put + and - on lipoma and + and – on parotid
Liquid retention	Thyroid/Thyroid
Lithiasis (stone-calculi-formation in organs or ducts) of gall bladder	Scapula/Scapula (*Mycobacterium lepra*) plus Gall bladder/Gall bladder (Virus reservoir)

Lithiasis of kidney (1)	Scapula/Scapula (*Mycobacterium lepra*) plus Kidney/Pomulus (*Plasmodium vivax* protozoa)
Lithiasis of kidney (2)	Pancreas Tip/Spleen (Common wart virus) plus Supra Spinal/Supra Spinal (Mycobacterium tuberculosis
Lithiasis of kidney (3)	Scapula/Scapula (*Mycobacterium lepra*) plus Pancreas Tip/Spleen (Common wart virus) plus Calyx/Ureter (Herpes 5)
Liver abscess	Liver/Left Kidney (Hepatic amoeba parasite—caused when amoeba go from pylorus to liver)
Liver flow obstruction	Esophagus/Esophagus (*Fasciolopsis buski* parasite)
Liver problems	Perihepatic/Perihepatic (*Morganella typhus* bacteria)
Liver problems, severe	Pylorus/Liver (Pinworm parasite)
Liver, extended	Subclavian/Subclavian (Diphtheria bacillus)
Loss, negative feelings from	Supraciliar/Rachidian Bulb (Special pair Vivian)
Lung congestion	Popliteal/Popliteal (*Pneumonia* bacteria)
Lung disorders	Canthus/Canthus (Aspergillus fungus); Hip/Hip (*Chlamydia pneumonia* bacteria) Humerus/Humerus (*Enterobacter pneumonia*); Scapula/Scapula (*Mycobacterium lepra* when it goes to lungs, produces emphysema); Subclavian/Subclavian (Diphtheria bacillus)
Lung infection, upper	Hepatic Ligament/Right Kidney (Adenovirus)
Lung problems relating to air conditioners	Cervical Plexus/Cervical Plexus (*Streptococcus fecalis* bacteria)
Lungs, blood in	Hip/Hip (Chlamydia pneumonia bacteria) associated with tuberculosis
Lungs, blood supply to	Temple/Temple
Lupus, false, with platelet alteration	Colon, Descending/Colon, Descending (*Enterobacter cloacae* bacteria) plus Vagina/Vagina (*Yersinia Pestis*) plus Gluteus/Gluteus (Intestinal parasites) plus Duodenum/Liver (*Chlamydia trachomatis* fungus)
Lupus, systemic erythematosus (SLE)	Renal Capsule/Renal Capsule (*Proteus mirabilis* bacteria) plus Sacrum/Sacrum (*Proteus mirabilis* bacteria) plus Pleura/Pleura (Viral pleuritis)

Lymph, flow alteration	Chiasm/Chiasm (Special pair Lucina)
Lymphatic ganglion inflammation	Hepatic Ligament/Right Kidney (Adenovirus)
Lymphocytes, T	Appendix/Thymus (Special pair Angeles)
Lysozyme toxin	Scapula/Scapula (*Mycobacterium lepra*)
Malaise, general	Thymus/Parietal (Rubeola virus)
Malassezia furfur --aggressive fungus	Tibia/Tibia
Malaria (*Plasmodium*) protozoan parasite (several species in Plasmodium parasite genus)	Cheekbone/Opposite Kidney (causes common tertian malaria); Parietal/Left kidney (*Plasmodium vivax*) giving tertian malaria; Hand/Hand, common malaria
Maltese fever	Spleen/Liver (*Brucella* bacteria)
Mange or scabies	Tongue/Tongue
Mange-like symptoms	Rectum/Adrenals (Leptospira): Hepatic Retro/ Hepatic Retro (*Toxocara* parasite)
Measles virus	Stomach/Adrenals
Measles (German—, 3-day measles)	Thymus/Parietal (Rubella virus)
Mediastinum, inflammation	Mediastinum, Inferior/Mediastinum, Superior (*Proteus mirabilis*)
Medication intoxication	Pylorus/Pylorus
Medulla damage	Eye/Eye (Cytomegalovirus); can cause paralysis
Megacolon	Colon, Transverse/Liver (Hepatitis G) plus Costal/ Liver (*Borrelia* bacteria) or Colon, Transverse /Bladder (*Vibrio cholera* bacteria) plus Ureter/Ureter (Varicella virus) plus Costodiaphragmatic/Costodiaphragmatic (*Trypanosoma cruzi* bacteria)
Melanoma	Brachial/Brachial (*Streptococcus* A bacteria)
Melanoma	See Cancer, skin
Meningitis, viral	Rachidian Bulb/Thyroid (*Meningococcus* virus) Meningitis by itself is not fatal, but if associated with Meningococcus virus, can be fatal.

Meningococcus bacteria	Dorsal/Lumbar
Menstrual pain	Kidney/Ureter (Special pair Machin); Pituitary/Ovary (Special pair Carmen)
Menstruation, suppression or absence of	Pituitary/Ovary (Special pair Carmen); Uterus/Uterus (Special pair Roberta)
Mental confusion	Jugular/Jugular (Tetanus); Kidney/Kidney (*Clostridium tetani* bacteria); Occipital/Occipital (Epstein-Barr virus); Parietal/Parietal (Encephalitis virus); Temporal/Temporal (*Typhus exanthematique* virus)
Mental retardation	Cerebellum/Rachidian Bulb (Newcastle virus)
Metastasis in cancer	Pleura/Pleura (Pseudomona aeruginosa bacteria) one side; Rectum/Rectum (Pseudomona aeruginosa bacteria)
Microsporum fungus	Radius/Radius; Knee Ligament/ Malleolus
Migraines	Temple/Temple (Special pair Isaac) plus Scapula/Scapula (Mycobacterium lepra); Temporal/Temporal (Typhus exanthematique virus)
Milk flow, not related to childbirth or nursing	Pituitary/Pituitary
Milk products, intoxication from	Stomach/Pylorus (*Perfringenes* bacillus) plus Liver/Liver (Hepatitis C)
Morganella typhus bacteria	Perihepatic/Perihepatic; Right Kidney/Liver
Motor disturbances	Kidney/Opposite Parietal; (Special pair Goiz)
Mouth problems, ulcers, bleeding, swelling	Angle/Angle (*Streptococcus fragilis* bacteria); Carina/Carina (Aphthous virus); Commissure/Commissure (Herpes 5 virus);
Mucus	Chondral/Chrondal (*Pneumocystis carini* fungus); Cranial/Cranial (*Anthrax* bacillus; Diaphragm/Diaphragm (*Candida albicans* fungus); Parietal/Parietal (Encephalitis virus)
Mucus in mouth or throat	Ulna/Ulna (Herpes 3)
Multiple Sclerosis	Deltoid, Middle/Deltoid, Middle (*Treponema palidum* bacteria) plus Pericardium/ Pericardium (*Staphylococcus aureus* bacteria) plus Eye/Eye (Cytomegalo virus); also check Medulla (in brain stem)

Multiple sclerosis, false	Cervical Plexus/Cervical Plexus (*Streptococcus fecalis* bacteria)
Muscular dyskinesia (impaired ability to make voluntary muscular movements)	Sciatic/Sciatic (Poliomyelitis virus)
Muscular insufficiency	Sciatic/Sciatic (Poliomyelitis virus)
Muscular problems in movement	Sacrum/Sacrum (*Proteus mirabilis* bacteria)
Muscular weakness	Parietal/Kidney (Goiz special pair)
Myasthenia gravis (tiredness/ weakness of muscles, beginning in face and throat, later, per-haps, breathing—most common in young women, old men)	Scapula/Scapula (*Mycobacterium lepra*) plus Cardia/ Adrenals (*Streptococcus* B bacteria) plus Fallopian Tube/Fallopian Tube (Parvo virus) plus Pancreas Tail/ Liver (*Clostridium botulinum*)
Mycobacterium lepra	Scapula/Scapula; the malignancy element in all cancers.
Mycobacterium tuberculosis	Supraspinal/Supraspinal
Myelocele, Myelomeningocele	Rectum/Rectum (*Pseudomona aeruginosa* bacteria) plus Dorsal/Lumbar (*Meningococcus* bacteria) plus Sacrum/ Sacrum (*Proteus mirabilis* bacteria)
Myoma, true non-cancerous uterine tumor	Scapula/Scapula (*Mycobacterium lepra*) plus Prostate/ Rectum (Papiloma virus) plus Counter caecum/ Countercaecum (*Bordatella pertussis* bacteria) plus Duodenum/Left Kidney (*Chlamydia trachomatis* fungus)
Nails, fungal infection	Rib/Rib (Onchomycosis)
Nasal disorders	Trachea/Trachea (Influenza virus)
Nasal polyps	Cranial/Cranial (*Anthrax* bacillus); Deltoid/Deltoid (*Treponema palidum* bacteria) plus Cranial/Cranial (*Anthrax* Bacillus) plus Paranasal Sinus/Paranasal Sinus (Viral sinusitis); Eyelid/Eyelid
Nasopharyngeal problems	Cranial/Cranial (*Anthrax* bacillus)
Neck ganglion, inflammation	Inguinal Nerve/Liver (Roseola virus); also check all Herpes viruses;

Neisseria catarrallis bacteria	Eyelid/Eyelid (can give nasal polyps)
Neisseria gonorrhea bacteria	Mandible/Mandible; 4th Lumbar/4th Lumbar;
Neocardia americana	Pre auricular/Pre auricular (can't open mouth)
Nephritis	Kidney/Kidney (*Clostridium tetani* bacteria)
Nephrotic Syndrome (1) (problems of protein in urine)	Duodenum/Left Kidney (*Chlamydia trachomatis* fungus) plus Colon, Ascending/Right Kidney (*Klebsiella pneumonia* bacteria) plus Calyx/Urethra (Herpes V)
Nephrotic Syndrome (2)	Pancreas Duct/Left Kidney (*Spirochete* bacteria) plus Gall Bladder Duct/Right Kidney (*Spirochete* bacteria) plus Kidney/Kidney (*Clostridium tetani* bacteria)
Nephrotic syndrome (3)	Liver/Right Kidney (Hepatic cirrhosis) plus Duodenum/Left Kidney (*Chlamydia trachomatis* fungus) plus Colon, Ascending/ Right Kidney (*Klebsiella pneumonia* bacteria)
Nerve cells	Check all Herpes virus locations, as herpes virus has a predilection for nerve cells
Nervous system	Rachidian Bulb/Thyroid (Meningitis virus); Sciatic/ Sciatic (Poliomyelitis virus)
Nervous system, central	Kidney/Opposite Parietal (See Goiz special pair)
Nervousness	Temporal/Temporal (Typhus exanthematique virus)
Neurofibroma (fiberlike growth of nerve tissue)	Perihepatic/Perihepatic (*Morganella typus*) plus Parietal/Parietal (Encephalitis virus) plus Mandible/ Mandible (*Niesseria gonorrhea* bacteria)
Neurological problems	Vagus nerve/Kidney of opposite side (Special pair); Occipital/Occipital (Epstein-Barr virus); Parietal/ Colon, Transverse (*Entamoeba histolytic* parasite)
Newcastle virus	Cerebellum/Rachidian Bulb (can be from improperly cooked chicken)
Nocturna, nycturia (urination, excess urination, especially at night)	Bladder/Bladder (*Streptococcus* G bacteria)
Nodules or bumps under skin	Ischium/Ischium (Oncocercosis parasite)
Norkwar virus	Sacrum/Femur

Nosebleed	Caecum/Caecum (*Trichomonas* parasite) Haemophylus influenza; Cranial/Cranial (Anthrax); Eye/Eye (Cytomegalovirus); Hip/Hip (*Chlamydia pneumonia* bacteria); Lachrymal/Lachrymal (*Klebsiella pneumonia* bacteria); Rachidian Bulb/Bladder (Hemorrhagic Dengue)
Obesity	Iliac/Iliac (Elena special pair); Thyroid/Thyroid
Onchocercosis volvulus parasite	Ischium/Ischium
Onchomycosis (any fungal infection of the nails)	Rib/Rib
Orf virus	Orbital Floor/Orbital Floor (skin disease from sheep)
Osteochondromatosis (non cancerous tumor of bone and cartilage)	Deltoid/Deltoid (*Treponema palidum* bacteria) plus Armpit/Armpit (Rabies virus) plus Inguinal Nerve/Liver (Roseola virus) plus Tibia/Tibia (*Malassezia furfur* aggressive fungus)
Osteomyelitis (bone, bone marrow infection) of lower extremities	Calcaneus/Calcaneus (*Rickettsia*) plus Tibia/Tibia (Malassezia furfur fungus) plus Hiatus/Testicle (*Helicobacter pilori* bacteria) plus Caecum/Caecum (*Trichomonas* parasite)
Osteoporosis	Parotid/Parotid (Special pair Lolita); Can also be helped with Parathyroid/Parathyroid (glandular dysfunction) involved in calcitonin secretion, giving calium to bones)
Osteosarcoma, lower limbs	Scapula/Scapula (*Mycobacterium lepra* bacteria) plus Calcaneus/Calcaneus (*Rickettsia*) plus Sciatic/Sciatic (Polio virus) plus Tibia/Tibia (Malassezia furfur fungus); of the knee: Scapula/Scapula (*Mycobacterium lepra* bacteria) plus Urethra/Urethra (Corona virus) plus Popliteal/Popliteal (*Pneumococcus* bacteria) plus Tibia/Tibia (*Malassezia furfur* fungus) plus Stomach/Pylorus (*Clostridium perfringens* bacteria giving metastasis)
Osteosarcoma, upper limbs	Scapula/Scapula (*Mycobacterium lepra* bacteria) plus Wrist/Wrist (*Rickettssia*) plus Ulna/Ulna (Herpes 3) plus Armpit/Armpit (Rabies virus)

Otitis	Eyelid/Eyelid (*Neisseria catarrallis* bacteria)
Otolaryngology disorders	Armpit/Armpit (Rabies virus)
Ovarian cyst	Fallopian tube/Fallopian tube (Parvo virus) plus Colon, Descending/ Colon, Descending (*Enterobacter cloacae* bacteria)
Ovary, dysfunction	Ovary/Ovary; Pituitary/Ovary
Over-activity in children	Supraciliar/Rachidian Bulb (Special pair)
Overweight from poor digestion of foods	Iliac/Iliac (Special pair)
Pain, abdomen	Countercaecum/Countercaecum (*Bordatella* bacteria)
Pain, arm	See pain, leg or arm
Pain, back	Cava/Cava (*Trycophyte* fungus) Trochanter, Major/Trochanter, Major (*Salmonella typhus* bacteria); Cava/Cava (*Trycophyte* fungus) Lower back: Achilles/Achilles (*Shigella* bacteria); Adrenal/Rectum (*Leptospira* parasite); Calcaneus/ Calcaneus (*Rickettsia*); Fallopian Tube/Fallopian Tube (Parvovirus); Inguinal Nerve/Inguinal (HIV 3 virus); Sciatic/Sciatic (Poliomyelitis virus); Ureter/Ureter (Varicella virus or chicken pox in adults); Hip/ Hip (*Chlamydia psittaci pneumonia*); Dorsal/Lumbar (*Meningococcus* bacteria); Sacrum/Sacrum (*Proteus mirabilis*); Testicle/Testicle (*Yersinia pestis*) plus / Fallopian Tube/Fallopian Tube (Parvovirus)
Pain, back of hand	Hand/Bladder
Pain, breast	Adrenal/Adrenal
Pain, chest	Adrenal/Adrenal
Pain, dorsal-lumbar	Deltoid, Middle/Deltoid, Middle (*Treponema palidum* bacteria)
Pain, elbow	Cervical/Dorsal (Special pair) Confused with tennis elbow.
Pain, Fallopian tube	Fallopian Tube/Ovary (can indicate ectopic pregnancy)
Pain, general	For specific or general pain, put negative magnet on pain area, positive on kidney of same side.

Pain, hip	Quadriceps/Quadriceps (insecticide or bismuth intoxication)
Pain, joints	Cheekbone/Opposite Kidney (*Malaria protozoan* parasite); Pituitary/Bladder (Dengue virus, common); check for syphilis in joints
Pain, kidney stone passing	Kidney/Ureter Special pair to ease pain
Pain, leg	Sciatic/Sciatic (Poliomyelitis virus)
Pain, leg or arm	Right Inguinal Nerve (+ pole)/Area of leg or arm pain (- pole)
Pain, muscular	Pancreas Tail/Liver (*Clostridium botulinum* bacteria)
Pain, neck	Cervical/Dorsal (Special pair)
Pain, nose	Cranial/Cranial (*Anthrax* bacillus)
Pain, pleura	Bladder/Bladder (Streptococcus G bacteria)
Pain, stomach	Colon, Transverse/Bladder (*Vibrio cholera* bacteria)
Pain, upper vs lower body	Wrist/Wrist (*Rickettsia* bacteria—upper) vs Calcaneus/Calcaneus (*Rickettsia* bacteria—lower)
Pain, waist	Quadriceps/Quadriceps (insecticide or bismuth intoxication)
Palpitation (pounding or racing of heart)	Sternocleidomastoid/Sternocleidomastoid (Nerve system dysfunction)
Pancreas	Parotid/Parotid (Lolita special pair); Differential Diagnosis: Pudendal/Pudendal or Parotid/Parotid (Parotiditis)
Pancreas Problems, differential diagnosis	Pudendal/Pudendal or Parotid/Parotid (Parotiditis)
Pancreatitis	Pancreas Body/Pancreas Tail (Special pair Ramses); Also check for botulism (Pancreas Tail/Liver) and a pair for false diabetes from Spirochete bacteria (Panceas Duct/Left Kidney)
Papiloma virus, often called cancer or pre cancer; confused with Parvo virus, corona virus or other viruses in same area	Anus/Anus; Prostate/Rectum
Paralysis	Sciatic/Sciatic (Poliomyelitis virus); Eye/Eye (Citamegalovirus)

Paralysis, diaphragm	Pineal/Rachidian Bulb (Guillan barre virus)
Paralysis, facial	Upper Ear/Upper Ear (Special pair) or Mastoid/ Mastoid (Filaria parasite)
Paralysis, weakness of members	Pineal/Rachidian Bulb (Guillan barre virus)
Paramoxivirus	Bladder Annex/Anus (Bladder Annex at ligament at side of bladder); gives gynological problems producing secretions, sweating
Parasites	*Balantidium typhus* *Cysticercus* *Entamoeba histolytic* *Enterobius vermicularis* *Fasciolopsis buski* *Filaria* *Giardia lamblia* *Hepatic amoeba* *Hookworm* *Intestinal amoebeasis* *Leishmania* *Leptospira* *Malaria protozoa* *Onchorcercosis vovulus* *Pinworm* *Plasmodium folisporum,* *Plasmodium vivax* *Scabies or mange* *Toxocara* *Toxoplasma gondii* *Triquina* *Trichomonas* *Trypanosoma brucei gambiense;* *Tripanosoma cruzi*
Parasympathetic nerves and headache	Cervical/Sacrum
Parathyroid disorders	Armpit/Armpit (Rabies virus)
Parathyroid disorders, differential diagnosis	See thyroid BMPs

Paratyphus bacteria	Trochanter, Major/Kidney
Pardoning or forgiving a grudge	Can relieve Poliomyelitis, according to Goiz
Parkinson's	Any bacteria in area of pancreas can be causal factor
Parotiditis virus	Pudendal/Pudendal (If in male, check also for Parotid/Parotid and if both pairs are present, can result in parotiditis, which can cause male infertility)
Parotid gland dysfunction, differential diagnosis	See Thyroid Gland Dysfunctions
Parotina, produced by parotid gland and pancreas	Parotid/Parotid (Lolita special pair)
Parrot fever	See *Chlamydia psittaci.*
Parvovirus	Fallopian tube/Fallopian tube
Pasteurela bacteria (giving Hepatitis A)	Colon, Descending/Liver
Pelvic disorders	Clitoris/Clitoris (*Spirochete* bacteria); Coccyx/Coccyx (Rotavirus); Popliteal/Popliteal (*Pneumonia* bacteria)
Pericardial cavity inflammation	Costodiaphragmatic/Costodiaphragmatic (Trypanosoma cruzi bacteria);
Pericarditis (inflammation of membrane around heart)	Appendix/Left Pleura; Pericardium/Pericardium (*Staphylococcus aureus coag+* bacteria)
Periodontal abscess	Mandible/Mandible (*Neisseria gonorrhea* bacteria) plus Angle/Angle (*Streptococcus fragilis*)
Personality changes	Interciliar/Rachidian Bulb (Special pair)
Pertussis bacillus	See Whooping cough
Pharynx problems	Angle/Angle (*Streptococcus fragilis* bacteria)
Phlebitis	Countercaecum/Countercaecum (Bordatella bacteria)
Phlegm	Chondral/Chondral (*Pneumosistis carini* fungus)
Photophobia	Cranial/Cranial (*Anthrax* bacillus)
Pinworm parasite (Enterobius vermicularis)	Pylorus/Liver (giving Hepatitis J)

Pituitary gland dysfunction, differential diagnosis	Cranial/Cranial (*Anthrax* bacillus); Eye/Eye (Cytomegalovirus); Pituitary/Bladder (Dengue, common); Parietal/Parietal (Encephalitis, viral); Malar/Sternum (Enterovirus); Caecum/Caecum, Lachrymal/Lachrymal (KIebsiella pneumonia bacteria); Rachidian Bulb/Thyroid (Meningitis, viral); Mandible/Mandible and/or Eyelid/Eyelid (*Neisseria* bacteria)
Pituitary tumors	Cranial/Cranial (*Anthrax* bacillus)
Pityrosporum fungus or *versicolor* or *Malassezia furfur*	Tibia/Tibia (Can produce a cancer when combined with another bacterium or virus.)
Plasmodium folisporum	1st Cervical/Pylorus
Plasmodium protozoa parasite	Hand/Hand; Parietal/Left Kidney
Plasmodium vivax	Cheekbone/Kidney (common malaria)
Pleural bleeding, disorders	Appendix/ Pleura of same side (*Staphylococcus aureus coag+* bacteria; Costal/Costal (*Proteus mirabilis*)
Pleuritis virus	Armpit/Armpit; Pleura/Pleura Two sides (vs Pleura/Pleura, one side, which is *Pseudomona aeruginosa* bacteria)
Pneumococcus or *Pneumonia* bacteria	Popliteal/Popliteal (Congestion in pelvis and/or lungs. Women with this pair, causing pelvic infection, often have same bacteria in lungs. Check both.)
Pneumonia	Colon, Ascending/Right Kidney (*Klebsiella pneumonia* bacteria); Check also for Goiz special pair, Parietal/Kidney.
Pneumonia, similar to	Pleura/Pleura (Pleuritis virus) two sides; Hip/Hip (*Chlamydia pneumonia* bacteria)
Pneumocystis carini fungus	Chondral/Chondral
Poisoning	Pancreas/Pancreas Heavy metal (often from sea food); Insecticides or bismuth: Quadriceps/Quadriceps; Medications: Pancreas/Pancreas; from powder (particles) of Teflon: Liver (back lobe)/ Left Kidney—special pair; Pylorus/Pylorous (medication intoxication)

Poisoning, protein (excess protein)	Pancreas/Pancreas (Ramses special pair)
Poliomyelitis virus	Sciatic/Sciatic; see pardoning
Polyoma virus	Left Temporal/Left Temporal (from aerosolized feces and urine from infected birds.)
Polyps	From union of a pathogenic virus and a pathogenic bacteria: Malar/Malar or Malar/Sternum (Enterovirus) plus Eyelid/Eyelid (*Neisseria catarrallis* bacteria)
Polyradiculo neuritis	Pineal/Rachidian Bulb (Guillan barre virus)
Potassium metabolism	Pancreas/Pancreas (See Ramses special pair)
Preemies, breathing problems from thorax tiredness	Temple/Temple and Scapula/Scapula
Pregnancy	Indicated by Uterus/Ovary (Duran special pair) If there is any chance of pregnancy, do not place magnets in the vicinity of the uterus and ovary at the same time.
Pregnancy, ectopic	Fallopian Tube/Ovary (With knowledge of polarity of gamete, can use opposite charge to push from Fallopian tube to uterus if done early enough in pregnancy.)
Pregnancy, false	Uterus/Uterus (Roberta special pair)
Prion reservoir	Right Temporal/Cardias –shelters prions
Proteus mirabilis bacteria--4 locations	Costal/Costal; Mediastinum, Superior/Mediastinum, Inferior; Renal Capsule/Renal Capsule; Sacrum/Sacrum
Pseudomona aeruginosa bacteria	Pleura/Pleura one side (vs. Pleura/Pleura, two sides, which is pleuritis virus.) Also Rectum/Rectum
Psoriasis	Bladder/Bladder (*Streptococcus* G bacteria) plus Brachial/Brachial (*Streptococcus* A) Also check Coronaria/Lung (*Streptococcus* A) plus Bladder/Bladder (Streptococcus G) plus Scapula/Scapula (*Mycobacterium lepra*); Tibia/Tibia (*Pityrosporum or versicolor or Malassezia furfur* fungus, which causes skin blotches that simulate psoriasis). Check also Tongue/Tongue (Scabies/mange);.

	Adrenals/Rectum (*Leptospira*); Thymus/Parietal (Rubeola measles); Ureter/Ureter (Chicken pox); Stomach/Adrenals (Measles—skin problems); and Supraspinal/Supraspinal (*Mycobacterium tuberculosis*)
Psoriasis (skin blotches), simulates	Tibia/Tibia (*Pityrosporum* or *versicolor* or *Malassezia furfur* fungus, which causes skin blotches that simulate psoriasis.
Psychological or pre psychotic disorders	Eyebrow/Eyebrow (Special pair); Pancreas/Pancreas (if from heavy metal poisoning)
Pterigium (non cancerous tumor within cornea)	Duodenum/Kidney (*Chlamydia trachomatis* fungus) plus Canthus/Canthus (Aspergillus fungus) plus Malar/Malar (Enterovirus)
Pterygoid, left (upper jaw)	Duodenum/Left Kidney (*Chlamydia trachomatis* fungus) plus Eye/Eye (Cytomegalovirus) &/or Malar/Malar (Enterovirus) plus Parietal/Colon, Transverse (*Entamoeba histolytic* parasite)
Pterygoid, right (upper jaw)	Duodenum/Left Kidney (*Chlamydia trachomatis* fungus) plus Eye/Eye (Citomegalovirus) or Malar/Malar (Enterovirus) plus Angle/Angle (*Streptococcus fragilis* bacteria)
Pulmonary degeneration	Scapula/Scapula (*Mycobacterium lepra*) plus Temple/Temple (Isaac special pair)
Pulmonary disorders	Costal/Costal (*Proteus mirabilis* bacteria); Dorsal 2/Dorsal2 (*Legionella* bacteria from air conditioners); Hiatus/Esophagus (*Enterobacter pneumonia* bacteria); Inferior Mediastinum, Inferior/Mediastinum, Superior (*Proteus mirabilis*); Parietal/Opposite Kidney (See Goiz special pair); Spleen/Duodenum (Special pair also giving leukemia);
Pulmonary fibrosis	Scapula/Scapula (*Mycobacterium lepra*) plus Dorsal/Lumbar (*Meningococcus* bacteria) plus Carina/Carina (Aphthous virus)
Pulmonary thrombus embolism	Scapula/Scapula (*Mycobacterium lepra*) plus Pleura/Pleura (Viral pleuritis) plus Dorsal 2/Dorsal2 (*Legionella* bacteria)

Quadriplegia from medullar lesions	Cervical Plexus/Cervical Plexus (*Streptococcus fecalis* bacteria give lesions)
Quadriplegia, common cause of	Pineal/Rachidian Bulb (Guillan barre virus) very contagious
R-40 virus (Replicating simian virus)	Colon, Sigmoid/Colon, Sigmoid (from end of colon in pelvis to beginning of rectum)
Rabies virus	Armpit/Armpit; in subclinical amounts, can seem like bipolarity; vaccinated animals can still transmit;
Ramsay Hunt syndrome (disease of facial and ear nerves, ear problems)	Pancreas/Pancreas (Toxic Pancreatitis) plus Esophagus/Esophagus (*Fasciolopsis buski* parasite) plus Trachea/Trachea (Influenza virus) plus Neck/Neck (*Blastocystis hominis* fungus). Also check for varicella zoster virus which causes shingles
Rashes	Wrist/Wrist or Calcaneus/Calcaneus (*Rickettsia* bacteria); Appendix/Tongue (Smallpox virus); Appendix/Right Testicle (rash that can affect prostate); Right Inguinal Nerve/Liver (Roseola); Stomach/Adrenal (Measles virus); Thymus/Parietal (Rubella virus); Ureter/Ureter (Shingles, Varicella or chicken pox virus)
Rattlesnake bite	Parietal/Parietal is helpful
Rectal bleeding	Duodenum/Left Kidney (*Chlamydia trachomatis* fungus) plus Hip/Hip (*Chlamydia pneumonia*)
Rectal mucus	Colon, Descending/Colon, Descending (Enterobacter cloacae)
Red blood cell number regulation	Sternum/Adrenals (Special pair)
Renal dysfunction	Kidney/Renal Capsule (same side, special pair); Bladder/Bladder (*Streptococcus* G bacteria); Parietal/Opposite Kidney (Goiz special pair)
Renal insufficiency	Parietal/Left Kidney (*Plasmodium vivax* protozoa) plus Liver/Right Kidney (Hepatic cirrhosis) plus Kidney/Kidney (*Clostridium tentani* bacteria) plus Renal Capsule/Renal Capsule (*Proteus mirabilis* bacteria); Perirenal/Perirenal (Bovine tuberculosis); can be confused with Urethra/Urethra (Corona virus)

Reovirus	Polygon/Polygon; Orbital floor/Orbital floor
Reservoir of bacteria, virus, fungi, parasites	Pleura/Pleura; Pleura/Peritoneum; Gall Bladder/Gall Bladder;Renal Capsule/Renal Capsule; Kidney/Renal Capsule; Inguinal Nerve/Inguinal Nerve; Trochanter, Lesser/Trochanter, Lesser; Stub/Stub (stub remaining after amputation of organ); Cardia/Temporal (special pair Boch, of prions); Subdiaphragm/Subdiaphragm (*Cysticercus* special pair Ecuador)
Respiratory problems	Diaphragm/Diaphragm (*Candida albicans* fungus); Hepatic Ligament/Right Kidney (Adenovirus); Humerus/Humerus (Enterobacter pneumonia). See also Breathing.
Retinitis pigmentosa (slow retinal degeneration leading to blindness; considered hereditary)	Paranasal Sinus/Paranasal Sinus (Viral sinusitis) plus Scapula/Scapula (*Mycobacterium lepra*) plus Subclavian/Subclavian (Diphtheria bacillus) plus Armpit/Armpit (Rabies virus) *Toxocara* parasite
Retro hepatic	*Toxocara* parasite giving mange-like symptoms
Rheumatic complications	Kidney/Pomulus (Gives malaria)
Rheumatic fever	Cardia/Adrenal (*Streptococcus* B)
Rheumatism, degenerative articular	Dorsal/Lumbar (*Meningococcus* bacteria) plus Mandible/Mandible (*Neisseria gonorrhea* bacteria)
Rheumatism, false	Deltoid, Middle/Deltoid, Middle (*Treponema palidum* bacteria); Quadriceps/Quadriceps (Special pair Magda)
Rhinitis	Lachrymal/Lachrymal (*Klebsiella pneumonia* bacteria); Trachea/Trachea (Influenza virus)
Rickettsia bacteria	Calcaneus/Calcaneus; Wrist/Wrist; (*Rickettsia* live as virus-like particles in cells of fleas, lice, ticks and mites and are transmitted to humans by bites from these insects and historically have caused many epidemics. The presence of both pairs, Calcaneus and Wrist, indicate Alzheimer's.)
Roseola virus	Inguinal Nerve/Liver (Common in children under three.)
Rotavirus	Coccyx/Coccyx

Rubella virus	Thymus/Left Parietal (Three-day measles)
Salmonella typhus bacteria	Trochanter, Major/Trochanter, Major (Typhoid Fever)
Salpingitis (inflammation of Fallopian tubes)	Fallopian Tube/Fallopian Tube
Scabies or mange parasite	Tongue/Tongue
Scarlatina in children	Bladder/Bladder (*Streptococcus* G bacteria)
Scarlatina, simulates	Tibia/Tibia (*Pityrosporum or versicolor or Malassezia furfur* fungus)
Scars, excess scar tissue	From excess of H+ ions. keloid Put + magnets on site.
Scorpion bite, to help pain	(same kind of poison as *Pneumococcus* and *Clostridium tetani*) Kidney/Kidney
Seizures	Ear/Ear (Toxoplasma gondii); Mastoid/Mastoid (*Filaria* parasite); Pancreas/Pancreas (Ramses special pair—use to stop seizures.)
Sexual overstimulation	Atlas/Atlas (Special pair)
Sexuality	Pineal/Pineal (Special pair) Put magnets horizontally.
Shigella bacteria (intestinal)	Achilles/Achilles
Shingles	Ureter/Ureter (Varicella zoster virus)
Sinus abscess	Esophagus/Esophagus (Influenza virus) plus Mediastinum/Mediastinum (*Proteus mirabilis* bacteria) plus Costal/Liver (*Borrelia* bacteria)
Sinus problems, chronic	Armpit/Armpit (Rabies virus)
Sinusitis, viral	Trachea/Trachea (Influenza virus); Forehead/Forehead;
Sinusitis, simulates	Eyelid/Eyelid (*Neisseria catarrallis* bacteria)
Skin cancer	Brachial/Brachial (Streptococcus A bacteria) plus Scapula/Scapula (*Mycobacterium lepra*)
Skin color, loss of	Ischium/Ischium (Onchocercosis)
Skin disease with blisters	Orbital Floor/Orbital Floor (Orf virus from sheep)
Skin problems	Brachial/Brachial (*Streptococcus* A bacteria); Scapula/Scapula (*Mycobacterium lepra*); Tongue/Tongue (Mange or scabies) Dermatitis type problems ; See also Rashes.
Skin, red coloration in	Tibia/Tibia (*Pityrosporum or versicolor or Malasssezia furfur* fungus)

Sleep disorders	Cervical/Cervical
Sleepiness, lethargy	Pancreas/Pancreas, from problem with potassium metabolism (see Ramses special pair)
Sleeping sickness	Parietal/Parietal (Encephalitis virus)
Smallpox	Appendix/Tongue
Sperm production	Hiatus/Right Testicle (*Helicobacter pilori* bacteria)
Sperm, lack of in semen (azoospermia)	Speen/Spleen (*Yersinia pestis* bacteria); Testicle/Testicle (*Yersinia pestis* bacteria); also Vagina/Vagina (*Yersinia pestis* bacteria)
Spina bifida	Dorsal/Lumbar (Meningococcus bacteria)
Spirochete bacteria	Clitoris/Clitoris; Gallbladder Duct/Right Kidney; Pancreas Duct/Left Kidney
Spirochete E bacteria	Clitoris/Pelvis
Spleen disorders, from fleas	Costodiaphragmatic/Costodiaphragmatic (*Trypanosoma cruzi* bacteria)
Spleen dysfunction	Spleen/Spleen (*Yersinia pestis* bacteria)
Spleen,differential diagnosis	See pancreas
Spondylitis, ankylosing (swelling,stiffness, and pain of vertebral joint in spine)	Deltoid, Middle/Deltoid, Middle (*Treponoma palidum* bacteria) plus Pericardium/Pericardium (*Staphylococcus aureus*) plus Quadrate/Quadrate (*Treponema palidum* bacteria) plus Stomach/Adrenal (Measles virus)
Staphylococcus albus bacillus	Epiploon/Epiploon
Staphylococcus aureus -	Pancreas Head/Liver giving Hepatitis K (No diagram given)
Staphylococcus aureus coag-	Pancreas Head/Adrenals
Staphylococcus aureus coag + bacteria (in air conditioners)	Pericardium/Pericardium; Appendix/Pleura
Staphylococcus epidermis	Mandible Branch/Mandible Branch (no diagram); Pancreas Head/Adrenals
Staphylococcus dorado cuag +	Pancreas Head/Adrenals
Sterility	Duodenum/Liver (*Chlamydia trachomatis* specialized bacteria living as a parasite); also see Fertility

Stomach dysfunction	Stomach/Stomach
Stomach infection	Ligament/Right Kidney (Adenovirus)
Stones – kidney, gallbladder	See lithiasis.
Streptococcus A bacteria	Coronaria/Left Lung; also Brachial/Brachial (skin problems)
Streptococcus B	Cardia/Adrenal; Cardia/Cardia (rheumatic fever, esophageal varices); Bursa/Elbow of same side;
Streptococcus C	Ischium Branch/Ischium Branch
Streptococcus fecalis bacteria	Cervical Plexus/Cervical Plexus
Streptococcus fragilis bacteria	Angle/Angle (mouth problems)
Streptococcus G bacteria	Bladder/Bladder
Stub	What is left of an excised organ; can be reservoir of virus, bacteria, fungi and/or parasite; depolarize over stump. See special pair Guadalupe. (Guadalupe special pair)
Sweating	Sternocleidomastoid/Sternocleidomastoid (Nerve system dysfunction)
Swine flu	Pancreatic ligament/Spleen plus Kidney/Kidney
Sympathetic nerve system dysfunction	Sternocleidomastoid/Sternocleidomastoid
Syncitial respiratory virus	Eyebrow/Eyebrow
Syphilis	Deltoid, Middle/Deltoid, Middle (confused with arthritis)
Syphilis bacillus	Quadrate/Quadrate (see also Deltoid, Middle)
Tailbone, degeneration, infection, irritation	Sacrum/Sacrum (*Proteus mirabilis* bacteria)
Tear secretion	Parietal/Parietal (Encephalitis virus)
Teeth falling out	Eyelid/Eyelid (*Neisseria catarrallis* bacteria)
Teflon intoxication	Liver posterior lobe/Left Kidney special pair
Tennis elbow	From lesion of long muscles of hand and/or arm. Use Cervical/Dorsal and also negative on injury, positive on same side kidney.
Testicles, problems of	Pudendal/Pudendal (Paroditis virus)

Tetanus—caused by bacteria-formed toxins of *Clostridium tetani*	Jugular/Jugular; Kidney/Kidney
Thirst	Pituitary/Rachidian Bulb (Diabetes insipid)
Thorax, muscular coordination	Cerebellum/Rachidian Bulb (Newcastle virus)
Throat problems	Cervical Plexus/Cervical Plexus (*Streptococcus fecalis* bacteria); Angle/Angle; Brachial/Brachial
Throat, chronic problems	Armpit/Armpit (Rabies virus)
Thrombocytopenic purpura, false	Colon, Derscending/Colon, Descending (*Enterobacter cloacae*) plus Bladder/Bladder (*Streptococcus* G) plus PancreasTip/Spleen (Common wart virus)
Thrush	Diaphragm/Diaphragm (*Candida albicans* fungus)
Thymus dysfunction	Thymus/Thymus
Thymus gland dysfunctions, differential diagnosis	Carina/Carina; (Aphthous virus); Diaphragm/Kidney (*Brucella abortus* bacteria); Diaphragm/Diaphragm (*Candida albicans* fungus); Humerus/Humerus (*Enterobacter pneumonia*); Index Finger/Index Finger (*Escherichia coli* bacteria); Esophagus/Esophagus (*Fasciolopsis buski* parasite); Hiatus/Right Testicle (*Helicobacter pilori* bacteria); Esophagus/Left side of Bladder (*Histoplasma capsulatum* fungus);Trachea/Trachea (Influenza virus); Armpit/Armpit, Pleura/Pleura (Pleuritis virus); Chondral/Chondral (*Pneumocystis carini* fungus) Costal/Costal, Renal Capsule/Renal Capsule, Sacrum/Sacrum, Mediastinum, Inferior/Mediastinum, Superior (*Proteus mirabilis* bacteria); Armpit/Armpit (Rabies virus); Thymus/Left Parietal (Rubella virus)
Thymus hormones	Thymus/Rectum (HIV 1) Affects production of thymus hormones (CD3,CD4 as well as T4 lymphocytes.)
Thymus, trapped, giving false AIDS	Mediastinum, Inferior/Mediastinum, Superior (*Proteus mirabilis*)
Thyroid	Parotid/Parotid (Lolita special pair)
Thyroid disorders	Armpit/Armpit (Rabies virus)

Thyroid gland dysfunctions, differential diagnosis	Carina/Carina (Aphthous virus); Cervical 3/ Supraspinal (*Balantidium typhus* parasite); Subclavian/ Subclavian (Diptheria bacillus); Humerus/Humerus (*Enterobacter pneumonia*); Tonsil/Tonsil (Herpes 2 virus); Trachea/Trachea (Influenza virus); Deltoid/ Kidney of same side (*Leishmania* parasite); Scapula/ Scapula (Leprosy bacillus); Tongue/Tongue, (Mange or scabies); Mandible/Mandible (*Neisseria gonorrhea* bacteria); Larynx/Larynx (Pertussis bacillus); Armpit/Armpit (Rabies virus); Cervical plexus/ Cervical plexus (*Streptococcus fecalis*); Angle/Angle (*Streptococcus fragilis*); Deltoid, Middle/Deltoid; also check Quadrate/Lumbar and Quadrate/Quadrate (*Treponema palidum* bacteria); Supraspinal/Supraspinal (*Tuberculosis* bacillus) Pudendal/Pudendal and Parotid/Parotid (Viral parotiditis)
Thyroxine, production of	Parotid/Parotid (Lolita special pair)
Tics, nervous	Ear, Upper/Ear
Tiredness	Kidney/Pomulus (Malaria); Parietal/Opposite Kidney (Goiz special pair); See Fatigue
Tongue cancer, false	Tongue/Tongue (Mange or scabies)
Tongue hemangioma (harmless tumor of massed blood vessels)	Tongue/Tongue (Mange or scabies) plus Subclavian Subclavian (Diphtheria bacillus) plus Esophagus/ Esophagus (*Fasciolopsis buski* parasite) plus Trachea/ Trachea (Influenza virus)
Toothache	Negative on tooth, positive on kidney of same side
Tosa (aphthous) virus	Carina/Carina
Toxocara parasite	Hepatic, Retro/Hepatic, Retro –mange-like symptoms
Toxoides (not virus or bacteria)	Nose/Nose
Toxoplasma gondii parasite	Ear/Ear
Trachea problems	Carina/Carina (Aphthous virus); Esophagus/ Esophagus (*Fasciolopsis buski* parasite)
Trachea-bronchial problems, often called "asthma"	Subclavian/Subclavian (Diphtheria bacillus)

Trauma	Adrenal/Adrenal; Kidney/Kidney
Treponema palidum bacteria	Deltoid, Middle/Deltoid, Middle Also check Quadrate/Lumbar, and Quadrate/Quadrate (Syphilis)
Trichomonas	Ileocecal Valve/Right Kidney; Caecum/Caecumn
Tricophyte fungus	Rib/Rib#1
Trycophyte fungus (very toxic)	Cava/Cava
Trypanosoma brucei gambiense	Iliac Crest/Iliac Crest; (African sleeping sickness with blood, kidney, and nervous system disorders
Trypanosoma cruzi parasite or Chagas disease	Costodiaphragmatic/Costodiaphragmatic; affects internal organs—heart, esophagus, colon—and peripheral nervous system
Tuberculosis	For abscessed lung: Supraspinal/Supraspinal (*Mycobacterium tuberculosis*) plus Esophagus/Esophagus (*Fasciolopsis buski* parasite) plus Dorsal 2/Dorsal 2 (*Legionella* bacteria); Check for tuberculosis in: Abdominal cavity; Bladder; Cerebrum; Fallopian tubes; Inguinal nerve; Joints; Kidneys; Lungs; Ovaries; Pericardium; Testicles; Fallopian tube
Tumor, vagina	Anus/Anus (Papiloma virus)
Tumors	Hepatic Ligament/Right Kidney (Adenovirus);
Typhoid Fever	Trochanter, Major/Trochanter Major (*Salmonella typhus* bacteria)
Typhus exanthematique virus	Temporal/Temporal
Typhus, common	Are in *Rickettsa* genus: Cervical3/Deltoid (*Balantidium typhus* parasite); Trochanter, Major/ Trochanter, Major (*Salmonella typhus* bacteria); Perihepatic/Perihepatic (Morganella typhus); Temporal/Temporal (Exanthematis typhus) .
Ulcers	Adrenals/Stomach (Measles virus)
	Hiatus/Right Testicle (*Helicobacter pilori* bacteria); Stomach/Adrenals (Measles virus)
Underactivity, lethargy and underdevolpment in children	Supraciliar/Rachidian Bulb

Ureteritis	Ureter/Ureter (Varicella virus or chicken pox in adults) Confused with Urinary Papiloma
Urethral disorders	Adductor/Adductor (HIV 2 virus)
Uric acid	See acid urine.
Urinary tract infections (dysuria)	See Goiz special pair
Urination, excessive, especially at night	Bladder/Bladder (*Streptococcus* G bacteria)
Uterine muscle tissue tumor (myoma), false	Colon, Descending/Colon, Descending (*Enterobacter cloacae* bacteria) plus Fallopian Tube/Fallopian Tube (Parvo virus) plus Ureter/Ureter (Varicella virus)
Uterus infections	Stomach/Pylorus (*Clostridium perfringens* bacteria)
Uterus, parasite in	Uterus/Uterus No danger to do this even in case of pregnancy, as it will just kill parasite but not cause abortion
Uveitis (swelling of uveal tract of eye)	Frontal/Frontal (Sinusitis virus) plus Nose/Nose (Toxoides—not virus or bacteria) plus Angle/Angle (*Streptococcus fragilis*)
Vaginal bleeding	Ureter/Ureter (Varicella virus or chicken pox in adults) Women who have had hysterectomies can still bleed with this. Also Hip/Hip (Chlamydia pneumonia bacteria)
Vaginal disorders	Adductor/Adductor (HIV 2 virus); Anus/Anus (Papiloma virus) Gives tumor growth in vagina.
Vaginal flux	*Countercaecum/Countercaecum* (*Bordatella bacteria*); Hip/Hip (*Chlamydia pneumonia* bacteria); Spleen/Spleen (*Yersinia pestis* bacteria); Testicle/Testicle (*Yersinia pestis* bacteria); Vagina/Vagina (*Yersinia pestis* bacteria)
Vaginal inflammation	Tensor/Tensor (*Giardinella vaginalis* bacteria)
Vaginal tumors	Anus/Anus (Papiloma virus)
Vaginal warts	Prostate/Rectum (Papiloma virus)
Varicella zoster virus	Ureter/Ureter (Chicken pox, shingles)

Varicose ulcers	Scapula/Scapula (*Mycobacterium lepra*) and from parasites;
Varicose veins,	If nerves in sacral area are aggravated by *Bordatella* bacteria, can cause varicosity; Countercaecum/Countercaecum; Iliac/Iliiac (Special pair)
Veillonella bacteria	Gluteus/Pylorus
Ventilation paralysis	Pineal/Rachidian Bulb (Guillan barre virus)
Vibrio cholera bacteria	Colon, Transverse/Bladder; Colon, Transverse/Liver (Hepatitis G)
Viral encephalitis virus	Parietal/Parietal
Viral hepatitis	Liver/Pleura
Viral meningitis`	See meningitis
Viral parotiditis	See parotiditis
Viral pleuritis	See pleuritis
Viral sinusitis virus	Nasal Sinus/Nasal Sinus
Viruses	Adenovirus
	Anasaki
	Aphthous
	Cytomegalovirus
	Cold, common
	Corona virus
	Coxsackie virus
	Dengue, common
	Dengue, hemorrhagic
	Epstein-Barr
	Encephalitis
	Distemper in puppies
	Enterovirus
	Guillan barre
	Hanta
	Hepatitis A,B,C. G
	Herpes 1,2,3,4,5 6
	HIV 1,3, 4, 5
	HTLV

	Influenza
	Intestinal
	Measles virus
	Meningococcus virus
	Newcastle
	Norkwar
	Orf
	Papiloma
	Paramoxivirus
	Parotiditis
	Parvo
	Pleuritis
	Poliomyelitis
	Polyoma
	R-40
	Rabies
	Reo
	Roseola
	Rubella (German measles)
	Small pox
	Syncitial respiratory virus
	Typhus exanthematique
	Varicella zoster (chicken pox)
	Viral encephalitis
	Viral hepatitis
	Viral sinusitis
	Wart virus, common
	Wart, vaginal
	Wart, pubic
Vision problems	Cranial/Cranial (*Anthrax*); Nose/Nose (Toxoides); Parietal/Parietal (Encephalitis virus); Liver/Liver
Vitiligio or hypochromia (acts on skin pigment)	Pineal/Pineal (magnets placed horizontally)
Voice, high in men	Testicle/Testicle (need to balance)

Vomiting	Achilles/Achilles (Shigella parasite)
Walk, uneven and staggering	Rachidian Bulb/Cerebellum (Newcastle virus)
Wart virus, common	Pancreas Tip/Spleen
Wart, flat	Tongue/Appendix (Smallpox virus) plus Bladder/Bladder (*Streptococcus* G)
Wart, vaginal	Prostate/Rectum (Papiloma virus)
Warts	Scapula/Scapula (Mycobacterium lepra) plus Thymus/Parietal (Rubeola virus)
Warts, pubic area	Anus/Anus (Papiloma virus) or Prostate/Rectum (Papiloma virus)
Weight gain	Parotid/Parotid
Weight loss	Iliac/Iliac (Elena special pair); Vagus Nerve/Vagus Nerve
White blood cells	Appendix/Thymus (affects immune system.) Also Spleen/Duodenum (Leukemia)
Whooping cough	Larynx/Larynx (*Bordatella pertussis* bacteria)
Wound	<u>General rule: Negative over wound, Positive on Kidney, same side</u> .To promote healing, close a wound: Nipple/Dorsal; To dry: Ureter/Ureter;
Yeast, giving anal symptoms	Liver/Anus
Yersinia pestis bacteria, intestinal	Flank/Flank
Yersinia pestis pneumonia	Goes to lungs and is very problematic, giving pneumonia; Latisimus/Latisimus (triangular muscle on back from scapula to hip)
Yersinia pestis bacteria	Spleen/Spleen
Yersinia pestis bacteria	Testicle/Testicle (similar to Ovary/Ovary, either of which can be in either men or women)
Yersinia pestis bacteria	Vagina/Vagina

DISCLAIMER

The biomagnetic pair information contained in the following section stems from the discovery and subsequent research of Isaac Goiz. The information is presented in partial fulfillment of Goiz's challenge in the year 2000 to his students to publicize his findings to the world, asking only that credit be always given to him for his discoveries.

The author is not a licensed physician and offers this information for educational purposes only. The author and publisher disclaim any liability or loss in connection with this information. The biomagnetic pairs themselves, as well as the drawings of their approximate location in no way intend to replace or substitute actual licensed medical evaluation and/or treatment. This publication is designed to educate and provide general information regarding the subject matter covered. However, laws and practices vary from state to state, country to country, and are subject to change. Because each situation is different, specific advice should be tailored to the particular circumstances. For this reason, the reader is advised to consult with his or her health adviser, and/or legal consultant about the specifics of the individual situation before continuing. All subsequent artist's renditions of the locations of each specific point of each biomagnetic pair are merely approximations and in no way constitute a precise location for each pair. The drawings are provided as a visual aid only, and by no means define a final locale for each point, or guarantee that the artists' renditions can be applied to every individual person. The drawings are of an average or generalized nature, and are not intended to represent scientific fact, *i.e.,* no multi billion dollar studies have been performed.

CLARIFICATION OF BMP COMPOSITION

Each biomagnetic pair that follows contains two separate point locations. Each point is represented in the Body Catalog by a Black Dot. Each biomagnetic pair contains two dots for two separate and opposite charges. The charges are not labeled as they may vary depending on the person and the location on the planet. One biomagnetic pair exists with one of the dots being **POSITIVE**, and the other being **NEGATIVE**. No biomagnetic pair exists with each of the two dots being the same charge. For that reason, the Body Catalog contains the locations of the points of each biomagnetic pair, but leaves the determining of which one of the points of the pair is **POSITIVE**, and which one is **NEGATIVE** and also the exact location of the points up to the energy artist doing the scanning.

For example, the pair COLON, TRANSVERSE/BLADDER, shows the location for the transverse colon to be right below the navel, and the location for the bladder on the right side of the bladder. Since the transverse colon is much bigger than represented by the dot in the drawing, it is up to the person scanning (the energy artist) to pinpoint the exact location on the transverse colon where the point is most accurately found (indicated by the greatest difference in heel lengths.)

The point location in this example for bladder is shown to be on the right side of the bladder, and should not be taken to be the only possible location for the biomagnetic bladder point location. The bladder point might also be found on the left side of the bladder and must be scanned for (moving the magnet) to locate the exact point on the bladder. So with the help of the pictures, we can see the approximate location of the two points of each biomagnetic pair, and in the actual scanning process, we can locate the absolute position. For that reason the scanning process is vital for optimum results.

CHAPTER 18
EXPLANTION OF BODY CATALOG OF
GOIZ BIOMAGNETIC PAIRS

Taking the example of "Neck," p. 177 of the Body Catalog of Biomagnetic Pairs, we see five different elements:

1➡NECK

2➡ Above the scapula on back by neck
But not on neck

3➡NECK/NECK

4➡Blastocystis hominis fungus

Goes to lung and radiates to
skin, bladder, and prostate

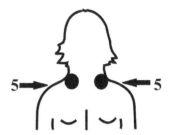

3➡ NECK/FEMUR

4➡ To kill all fungus

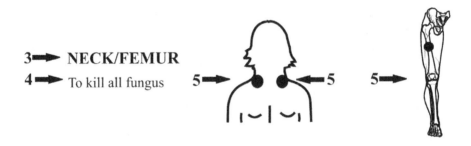

<u>Explanation</u> The five elements are separated in the following manner. (Learn more from pp. 61-3 of the book and the discussion and scanning video on our website: (www.bioen-ergeticbasics.com)

1. IN **BOLD** LETTERS, THE NAME OF BIOMAGNETIC POINT
2. LOCATION OF BIOMAGNETIC POINT
3. IN CAPITAL LETTERS, NAME OF BIOMAGNETIC PAIR
4. NAME OF PATHOGEN OR DYSFUNCTION AND PERTINENT INFORMATION ABOUT BIOMAGNETIC PAIR
5. MAGNET PLACEMENT FOR EACH BIOMAGNETIC PAIR: NEGATIVE AND POSITIVE SITES TO BE DETERMINED IN SCANNING

BODY CATALOG OF GOIZ
BIOMAGNETIC PAIRS

DISCLAIMER:

The biomagnetic pair information contained in this section stems from the discovery and subsequent meticulous research of. Isaac Goiz . The author is not a licensed physician and offers this body catalog as an educational and research tool only. These illustrations are schematic in nature and to locate exactly the point of greatest polarization of an organ, moving the magnet around on the organ is suggested. Please refer to color illustrations with scanning points at the beginning of the book.

ACHILLES
Between ankle and knee, posterior

ACHILLES TENDON/ACHILLES TENDON
Shigella bacteria can be from
dirty water as found in ice treats, ice cream,
cheeses, swimming pools, etc.

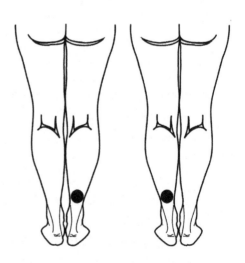

Gives diarrhea, vomiting,
Intestinal gas; headache
itching in groin.

ADDUCTOR

On inner surface of upper thighs

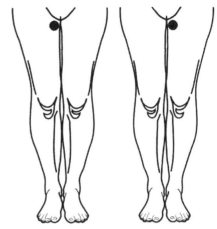

ADDUCTOR/ADDUCTOR

HIV 2 virus

Not true AIDS, as it does not affect thymus

Gives urethral and vaginal disorders
in women

ADRENALS

At bra height on back

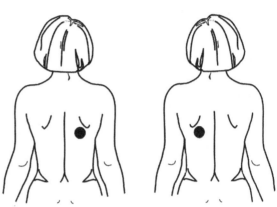

ADRENAL/ADRENAL

Glandular dysfunction

Patient has suffered trauma.

Addison's disease with swelling,

chronic fatigue, inability to

respond to infections

chest/breast pain

ADRENALS/ALL OVER FRONT OF BODY

Not a regular pair but a syndrome: a
biomagnetic pathology.

(The whole front of body is positive and the
adrenals are negative, so just put the
positive magnet on any place on front of
body that checks out as positive and the negative
magnet on the adrenals to get rid of the
symptoms)

Is true allergic asthma; rare.

(False asthma can come from other
things like rabies, etc)

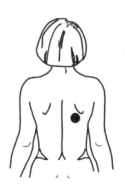
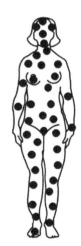

ADRENALS/RECTUM

Leptospira parasite
Can be confused with
Meningococcus
Is similar to mange. Transmitted
by animals
Gives disturbances
in breathing pathways,
mucus in digestive tract
Flatulence in rectum

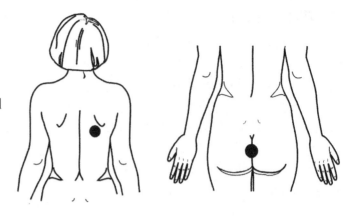

ADRENALS/STOMACH

Measles virus
In a child is rather light, but in the
adult it always manifests with
high alimentary canal bleeding
and can give ulcers
Main cause of gastritis (together with
helicobacter pilori) One woman got
measles from eating infected eggs.

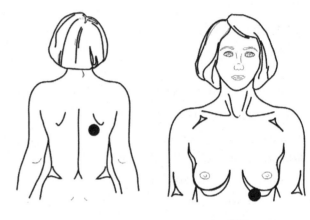

ALVEOLUS

Above heart at armpit height

ALVEOLUS/ALVEOLUS

Help respiratory process of
allowing oxygen to move into
blood, carbon dioxide to be
removed from blood.

ANGLE

Corner angle of mandible

ANGLE/ANGLE

Streptococcus fragilis bacterium

Mouth and pharynx problems

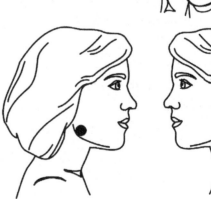
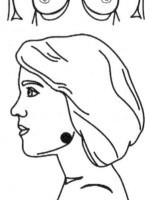

Ulcers, bleeding, swelling of mouth
This pair contributes to dental caries.
(Goiz thinks caries is a combination
of causes, as are all degenerative
problems)

ANUS
At end of tailbone
at sides of intergluteus fold

ANUS/ANUS
Papiloma virus
Put magnets at anus, horizontally,
Side by side

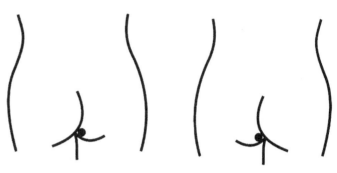

Gives tumor growth in vagina in women,
Warts in pubic area
Not common in men
Also check Prostate/Rectum

ANTIPOLE
Posterior to poles

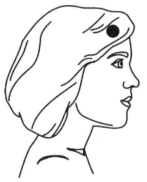
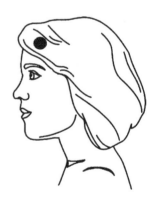

ANTIPOLE/ANTIPOLE
Aerobacter aeruginosa bacteria,
one of main causes of
cranial tumors

APPENDIX
Lower right abdomen; extends
downward from caecum.

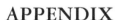

APPENDIX/PLEURA of the same side
Staphylococcus aureus cuag+ bacteria
Larynx, trachea, pleura disorders
Main cause of pleural bleeding

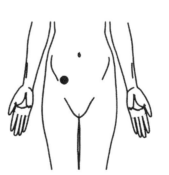
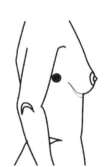

APPENDIX/PLEURA of left side
Gives Pericarditis (see "pericardium")

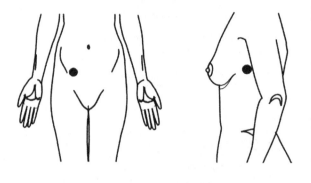

APPENDIX/THYMUS
Is Special pair Angeles
This raises or influences the capacity
of the immune system, involves
T lymphocytes and white
blood cells

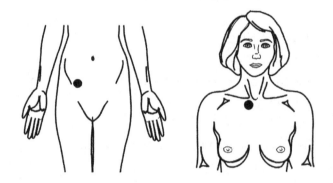

APPENDIX/TONGUE
Smallpox virus

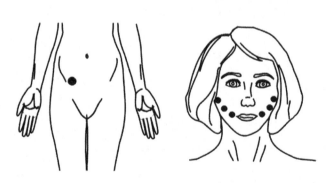

APPENDIX/RIGHT TESTICLE
A rash that can affect prostate

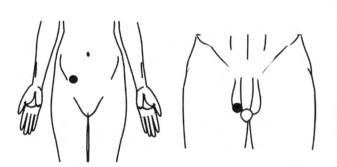

ARMPIT
Underarm

ARMPIT/ARMPIT
Rabies virus
Pleuritis virus
Otolaryngology disorders, throat and
chronic ear problems, sinus problems,
asthma, parathyroid and thyroid disorders,
irritability, chronic cough, eye irritations,
headaches

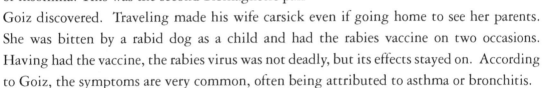

Get new toothbrush, lipstick, razor,
hair brush, comb, and washcloths
and sponges for bathing. Try this pair in cases
of insomnia. This was the second biomagnetic pair
Goiz discovered. Traveling made his wife carsick even if going home to see her parents.
She was bitten by a rabid dog as a child and had the rabies vaccine on two occasions.
Having had the vaccine, the rabies virus was not deadly, but its effects stayed on. According
to Goiz, the symptoms are very common, often being attributed to asthma or bronchitis.

ATLAS
On strong bone at back and
above base of skull—at first vertebra
where head turns—at level of lower
part of ear

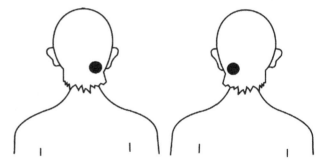

ATLAS/ATLAS
Special pair Juana
Use horizontal magnet pairs

Regulates sexual libido, frigidity, lack of
or presence of sexual feelings

AURICULAR, pre

In front of ear

PRE AURICULAR/PRE AURICULAR

Neocardia Americana
(can't open mouth)

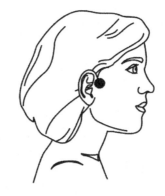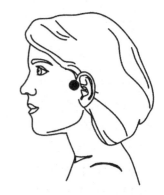

BLADDER

Below uterus put magnets horizontally
on each side of bladder.

BLADDER/BLADDER

Urinary incontinence, *Streptococcus*
G bacterium Pleura pain, renal problems,
scarlatina in children, Nocturia in adults
Combined with *Streptococcus* A it gives
psoriasis (which, says Goiz, "Is not psychosomatic and is
transmitted through cuts or bites")

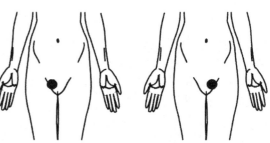

BLADDER ANNEX

At ligament side of bladder

BLADDER ANEX/ANUS

Gives gynecological problems
producing secretions, sweating.

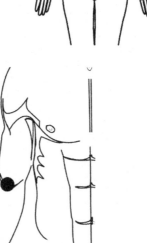

BRACHIAL

At inner bend of elbow by
brachial muscle

BRACHIAL/BRACHIAL

Streptococcus A bacteria

Gives skin problems, dermatitis,
melanoma, and allergies.

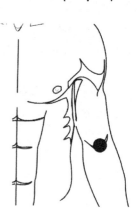

If combined with *Streptococcus* G, can give
psoriasis, which can be confused with cancer.
If combined with leprosy, gives skin cancer.

This pair can give problems of high cholesterol
leading to coronaries, as the cholesterol can
block entrance to heart. Depolarizing this
pair can help high cholesterol, says Goiz.

BURSA
At crease between deltoid and
bone where arm joins trunk of body

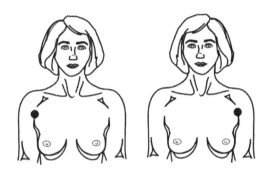

BURSA/BURSA
Actinomyces bacteria, anaerobic
filamentous bacteria
Occurs especially in women
Who have an IUD in place

CAECUM
The blind pouch in which the large intestine
begins and into which the ileum opens on
one side

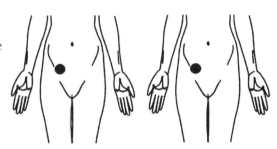

CAECUM/CAECUM
Haemophilus influenza
Trichomonas parasite.
Alters vasentarity

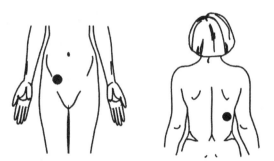

CAECUM/RIGHT KIDNEY
Pair for *Klebsiela pneumonia*

CALCANEUS

Large heel bone
Put magnets on back part of foot.

CALCANEUS/CALCANEUS

Rickettsia bacteria from dog or cat
Inflammation symptoms can be located
from navel down to heel
Pain in lower body
Can give false symptoms for
Alzheimer's. If person tests positive
for Calcaneus/Calcaneus and Wrist/Wrist,
that is true Alzheimer's (which Goiz
describes as "intoxication from something
very toxic").

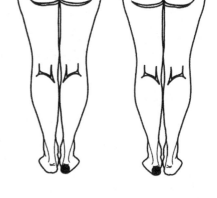

CALYX

A calyx is the cup-shaped structure
in the kidneys formed from the
branching of the renal pelvis.
It covers tips of medullar pyramids and
collects urine

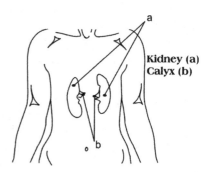

CALYX/URETER

Herpes 4.
Affects blood pressure

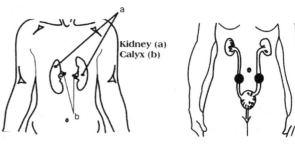

CANTHUS

Outer corner of eye

CANTHUS/CANTHUS

Aspergillus fungus
Affects eye and lungs and

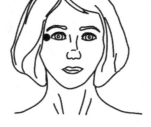
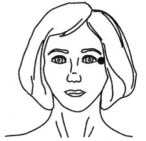

kidneys, can cause immune deficiency
Main cause of glaucoma and other eye problems.
For conjunctivitis, treat with Canthus/Canthus
plus Hepatic Ligament/Right Kidney

CARDIA
Connects esophagus and
stomach, under mediastinum at
5th vertebra (at normal bra level)

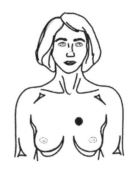
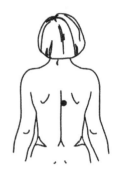

CARDIA/ADRENAL
Streptococcus B
disorders at height of cardia
Gives rheumatic fever and
esophageal varices

CARDIA/MASTOID
Plus Mediastinum/Mediastinum
Yields a hiatus hernia

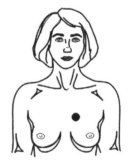
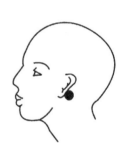

CARINA
At height of breasts on each side
of sternum (where trachea divides
into two, on inner side of each nipple)

CARINA/CARINA
Aphthous virus
Aphthous fever
Transmitted by milk products
Mistaken for AIDS, and is
confused with Herpes 3 and 4
Very common
Produces sores in mouth, bronchial
and tracheal symptoms

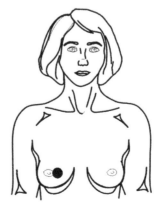
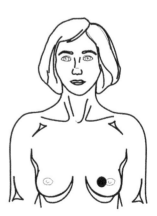

CAROTID
On side of neck by carotid artery

CAROTID/CAROTID
Special pair Marimar (daughter of Prada)
Changes arterial hypertension

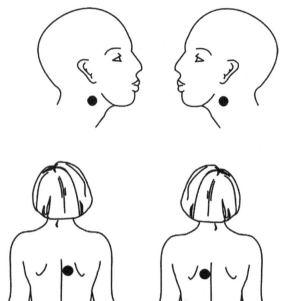

CAVA
At vena cava above adrenals
By spine and lower tip of shoulder blade

CAVA/CAVA
Trycophyte fungus
Back pain
Is terribly toxic
Can give fungal problems
at feet
Usually need antifungal remedy in
addition to depolarization

CEREBELLUM
Above rachidian bulb

CEREBELLUM/CEREBELLUM
One magnet above
another.
For convulsive crises.

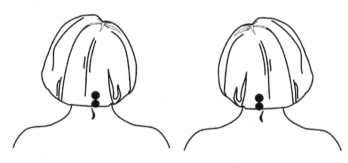

CERVICAL
On back of neck

CERVICAL/CERVICAL
Sleep disorders (Also see Rachidian
bulb/Rachidian bulb for insomnia)

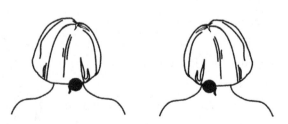

CERVICAL/DELTOID
Balantidium typhus
Causes serious diarrhea
See also Cervical/Supraspinal

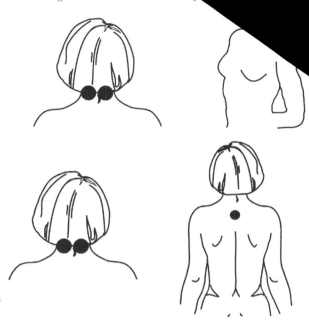

CERVICAL/DORSAL
Special pair Pasciano
For elbow pain, carpal tunnel
Put one magnet on neck, the other
directly below it
"This pair," says Goiz, "is in the last
cervical vertebra and the first dorsal
one and is responsible for sharp pain in
neck and elbow, not to be confused
with tennis elbow, which comes from a lesion of the long one supinator muscle on the
hand." Magnets here can help all if these problems.

CERVICAL/SACRUM
Parasympathetic nerves
Problems of headache in women
If there are bacteria or viruses
present in glands, can affect glands
Putting magnets on area can
regulate glandular disorders

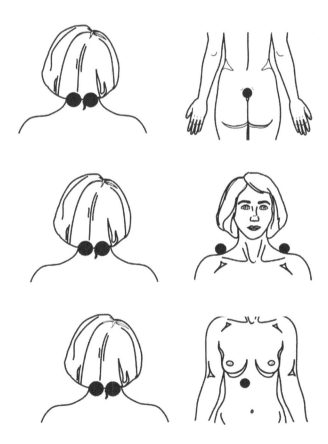

CERVICAL/SUPRASPINAL
Balantidium typhus parasite

1ˢᵗ CERVICAL/PYLORUS
Neurological involvement

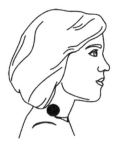
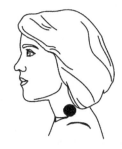

...US

... neck at 45° angle

.../CERVICAL PLEXUS

...cteria

Usually ... with air conditioners
and gives probl...ns in throat and lungs
Gives bronchial problems

False multiple sclerosis, it infiltrates in the medullar cord and makes lesions on the medulla producing quadriplegia

CHEEKBONE
Bone of cheek. Scan both cheekbones.

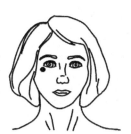
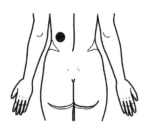

CHEEKBONE/OPPOSITE KIDNEY
Malaria protozoan parasite
Same as fibro myalgia—many cases in
New York and Canada
Pain in all joints (Could also be syphilis. Check.)

CHEEKBONE/KIDNEY
Plasmodium vivax protozoa parasite
Causes common tertian malaria

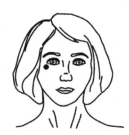
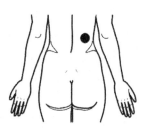

CHIASM
In middle of temporal
behind temples

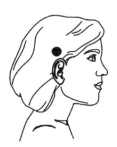
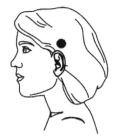

CHIASM/CHIASM
Special pair Lucina
Regulates flow of lymph
and as such can cause lymphatic flow problems if polarized. Can occur as result of infection or trauma.

CHIN

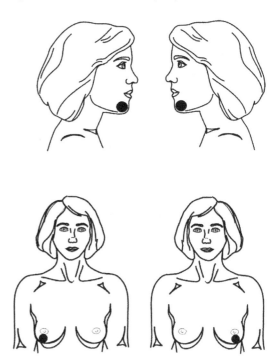

CHIN/CHIN
Herpes 8.

CHONDRAL
Below nipples

CHONDRAL/CHONDRA.L
Pneumocystis carini fungus

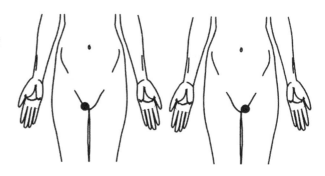

Manifests in lung with chronic cough, phlegm, chronic bronchitis

CLITORIS
Anterior portion between labia minor
Middle of pudendal area

CLITORIS/CLITORIS
Spirochete bacteria
Pelvic disorders

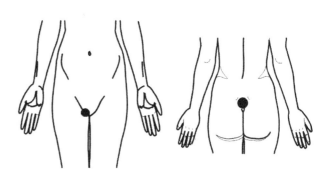

CLITORIS/SACRUM
Spirochete E
Relapsing fever, skin problems

COCCYX

Check various points around end of
tailbone, a little above anus. Is vertical
with magnets one above another.

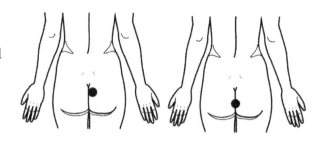

COCCYX/COCCYX

Rotavirus
Pelvic disorders

COLON, ASCENDING

A little more inside than duodenum

ASCENDING COLON/
DESCENDING COLON

Herpes 1 virus
Associated with varicella (chicken pox)
Faja de la reina

ASCENDING COLON/LIVER

Klebsiella bacteria (Hepatitis E)

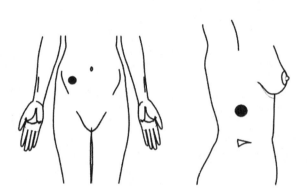

ASCENDING COLON/RIGHT KIDNEY

Klebsiella pneumonia bacteria
Gives pneumonia

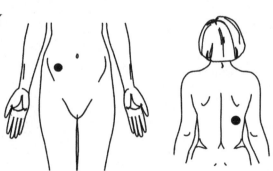

COLON, DESCENDING
Below waist at left side

DESCENDING COLON/DESCENDING COLON
Enterobacter cloacae
Transmitted by mucus from dogs, cats,
and farm animals
Prolapsed bladder or colitis,
gives digestive problems, gas, poor
absorption, distends lengthwise the
descending colon and displaces all else to
the other side of the abdomen
In women, can perforate organs and go into rectum, causing hemorrhoids or rectal mucus.
Is helped with bismuth.

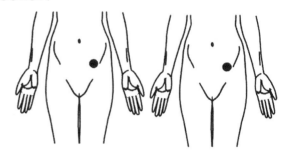

DESCENDING COLON/LIVER
Hepatitis A
From *Pasteurela* bacteria
Hepatitis E; Hepatitis G

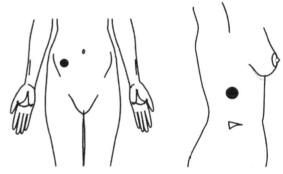

DESCENDING COLON/ RECTUM
Is special pair Olazo (an engineer from
Orizaba, Mexico)
For obstruction of the intestine.
Can stop intestinal blockage
and constipation

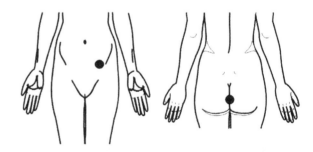

COLON, SIGMOID
The part of the colon that extends from
the end of the colon in the pelvis to the
beginning of the rectum

SIGMOID COLON/RECTUM
R-40 virus
Symptoms: somnolence, stupor, coma

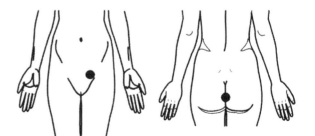

COLON, TRANSVERSE
Hanging below navel. Search for it.

TRANSVERSE COLON/BLADDER
Vibrio cholera bacteria
Cholera: Stomach pain, diarrhea,
headache, dehydration, constipation.
Supposedly there is no cholera, but
it is found in developed countries
in less pronounced form.

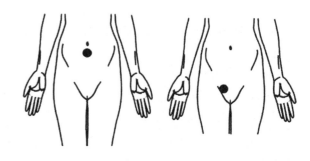

TRANSVERSE COLON/ LIVER
Hepatitis G

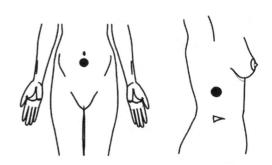

COMMISSURE
Point where upper and lower lips meet

COMMISSURE/COMMISSURE
Herpes 5 virus. Cold sores.

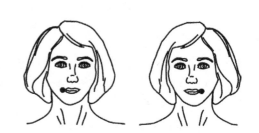

CORONARIA /RIGHT LUNG
Coronaria is above the left breast and
heart--near shoulder--and right lung
Streptococcus A bacteria
Provokes heart attacks
With *Streptococcus* A +
Streptococcus G = psoriasis.

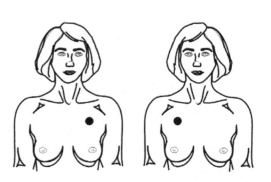

COSTAL

At height of ribs joining
Base of sternum, bilateral
Forward of underarms towards outer
edge of breast

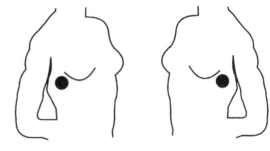

COSTAL/COSTAL

Proteus mirabilis
Pleural, pulmonary and diaphragm
manifestations

COSTAL/LIVER to HEPATIC DUCT

Borrelia bacteria
Is deadly
Is like *Trypanozoma*.
Main cause of mega colon (if in combination
with *Vibrio cholera*)

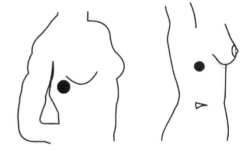

COSTODIAPHRAGMATIC

Under and in front of left armpit at level of
diaphragm (below pancreas tail) Put
magnets horizontally side by side

COSTODIAPHRAGMATIC/
COSTODIAPHRAGMATIC

Trypanosoma cruzi bacteria or Chagas disease
Transmitted by fleas
If it goes to pancreas,
can give false diabetes
Affects heart and spleen
If it reaches stomach, can give
gastric insufficiency
Common in Mexico
6,000 people die/ year of this in Central America.
Gives severe cardiovascular problems,
hypertension due to organ blockage
"Relieve organ blockage and hypertension

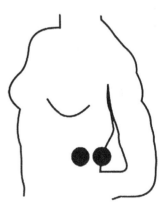

disappears," say Goiz.

Cardiopathy or cardiac insufficiency, inflamed pericardial cavity

One of main causes of arrhythmia of heart

COUNTER CAECUM

Is name of body area on left, opposite or as a mirror image of caecum on right (at head of femur)

COUNTER CAECUM/COUNTER CAECUM

Bordetella bacteria

Comes from fruits and vegetables

Gives problems, pain in abdomen,

One of main causes of vaginal flux—producing rectal and vaginal mucus in women

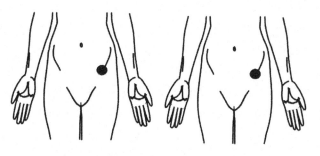

Diarrhea, digestive problems

Can cause phlebitis

If nerves in sacral area are aggravated, varicose veins result

Disease of head of femur, can destroy it, resulting in a hip surgery; Atherosclerosis involvement

CRANIAL

At top of nose

CRANIAL/CRANIAL

Bacillus anthrasis

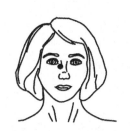
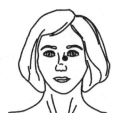

Nasopharyngeal problems, nasal polyps, pain, bad vision, photophobia, mucus, cysts, hypophyseal tumor

DELTOID, MIDDLE
Near top of shoulder

MIDDLE DELTOID/ MIDDLE DELTOID
Treponema palidum bacteria
If one has this, also check Quadrate/Lumbar
Syphilis.
Is confused with arthritis
Gives false articular rheumatism
Is from vaginal or urethral transmission,
Not necessarily sexual
Gives dorsal-lumbar pain

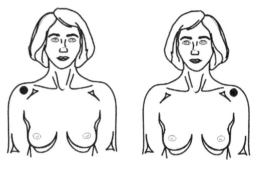

DELTOID/ KIDNEY OF SAME SIDE
Leishmania parasite
From sand fly bite
Skin sores, fever, spleen damage

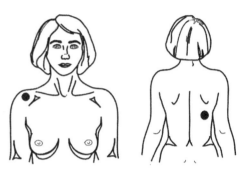

DIAPHRAGM
Is muscle dividing the abdominal and
chest cavity. A little below esophagus,
horizontally

DIAPHRAGM/ DIAPHRAGM
Candida albicans fungus
A fungus is an opportunist; is
transmissible from spores
There is a virus behind it!
Thrush
Mucus, respiratory diseases

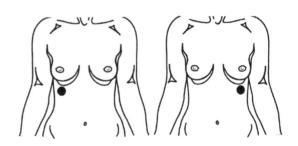

DIAPHRAGM/KIDNEY
Brucella abortus bacteria
excites peritoneum and miscarriage can occur
Impact with magnets on same side.

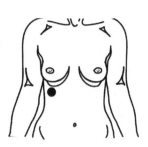 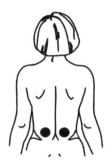

DIAPHRAGM HOLE/DIAPHRAGM HOLE
At center of diaphragm

Giardia lamblia
Gives severe digestion problems.

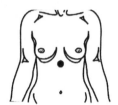 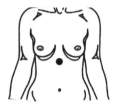

DORSAL
Shoulder blade height on spine

DORSAL 2/DORSAL 2
Legionella bacteria
Pulmonary problems
Transmitted by air conditioners and
air on planes

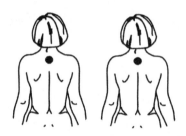

DORSAL/ LUMBAR
Meningococcus bacteria
Put one magnet between shoulder blades,
one at waist
Gets established in medullar tube or meningocele
Causes alterations in meningocele,
melocele, & meningomielocele
Spina bifida
If associated with gonococcus it
produces deforming rheumatoid arthritis,

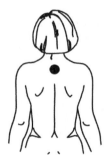 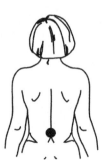

Arthritic rheumatism. Cartilaage destroyed with gonococcus, which produces lysozyme toxin, giving rheumatoid arthritis.

DUODENUM
Right edge of pelvis

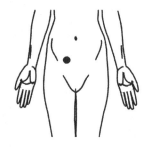 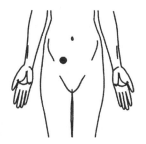

DUODENUM/DUDENUM
Duodenal dysfunction
Nervous colitis, irritable
colon, since food ferments
in colon

DUODENM/LEFT KIDNEY
Chlamydia trachomatis fungus
Is main cause of cervical-uterine cancer if
associated with
Pseudomona or *Yersinia,* giving false cancer.
From dirty water or sex--one of most
common sexually transmitted diseases
in North America. Gives lesions in eye,
pterygiums (corpulence in front of eye)
related to Enterovirus; also gives lesions in
lining of urine passage (urethra) and lower end
of uterus(cervix).(Chlamydia, gonorrhea, and syphilis
are entering the USA via Mexican and Central
American immigrants.)

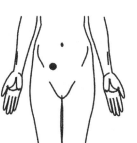 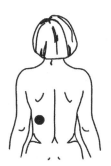

DUODENUM/RIGHT KIDNEY
Diabetes mellitus
The only true diabetes

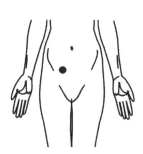 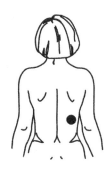

DUODENUM/SPLEEN
Leukemia
Is confused with brucellosis.

DUODENUM/LIVER
Hepatitis D virus.

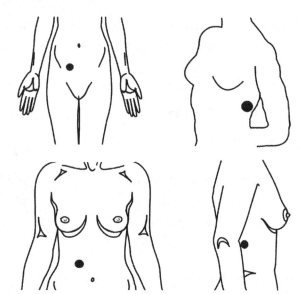

EAR
Over ear canal

EAR/EAR
Toxoplasmosis parasite
Produces repeated convulsions
Caused by the toxoplasma
Gondii
Spread by cat and bird feces
Harmful to pregnancy

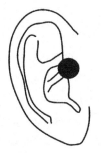
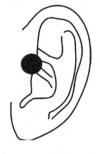

Depolarizing here can help correct
problems of horizontal equilibrium
(For vertical equilibrium, see Pole/Pole)

EAR/OPPOSITE KIDNEY

Special Pair Goiz
This is the second place to check
(Goiz special pair) if
Parietal/Kidney gives no results

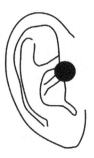
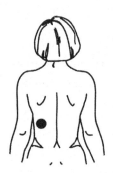

EAR, UPPER

Over auricular cartilage

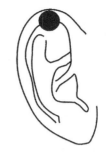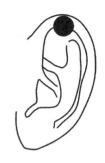

UPPER EAR/UPPER EAR

Leni special pair

Regulates cranial pairs of brain

Produces intoxication, Gives nervous tics

For facial paralysis if not from mastoid

Can improve hearing

ELBOW

On elbows, outer pointed part

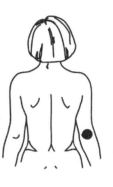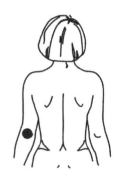

ELBOW/ELBOW

Is special pair Castaneda

Eye dysfunctions

EPIPLOON

At sides of bellybutton, both magnets right or both left, vertically

This produces a charge in the pancreas

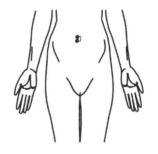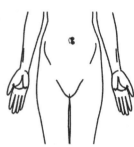

EPIPLOON/EPIPLOON

Staphylococcus albus bacillus

Gives common acne

ESOPHAGUS

At side of trachea on left side

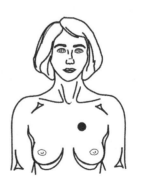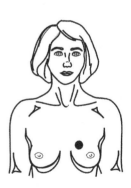

ESOPHAGUS/ESOPHAGUS

Fasciolopsis buski parasite or

Hepatic faciola gives false cancer,

tracheal, digestive, cardiac problems.

Obstructs normal flow in liver,

Gives hyporexia, bulimia, anorexia from lack

of appetite *Fasciolopsis buski* is a snail found in water, watercress, etc.

ESOPHAGUS/LEFT (side of) BLADDER
Histoplasma capsulatum fungus
Fungus goes directly to lung

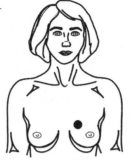 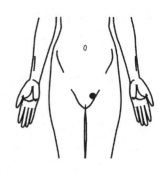

EYE
Whole eye

EYE/EYE
Cytomegalovirus
Good for painful muscles
Nervous system diseases such as M.S.
(Some patients diagnosed with
M.S. don't actually have M.S.,
which, says Goiz, must
involve Eye/Eye + the medulla)

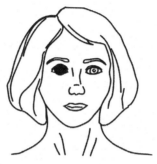 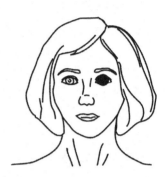

Attacks spinal medulla and produces
Multiple sclerosis when associated
with another pathogen,
Is curable as long as no medulla
Damage exists
(You can leave a magnet on eye
all night long and no harm will occur.)

EYE/EYELID
Can have two signs (+ and -) in one
location (such as right eye, right eyelid)
or one on each side as shown
Gives false AIDS

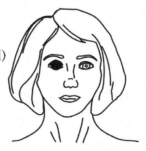 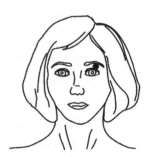

EYEBROW

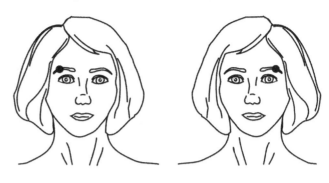

EYEBROW/EYEBROW
Syncitial respiratory virus
Psychological or pre-psychotic
disorders
Makes a rug-like
Structure of cells hooked
Together, affecting
respiratory system.

EYELID

At highest point of eyelid,
just below brow

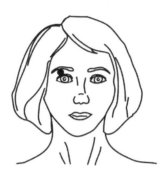
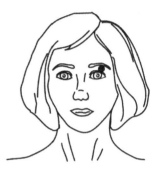

EYELID/EYELID
Neisseria catarrallis bacteria

If combined with gonorrhea, teeth
fall out.
Gives gingivitis and otitis.
Confused with sinusitis.

FALLOPIAN TUBE

On edge of bladder

FALLOPIAN TUBE/FALLOPIAN TUBE
Parvovirus
Salpingitis = inflammation of Fallopian tube.
Produces infertility, irritability
Points are separated if she has
had a baby,close together if not.
In a male, points are close together.
Parvovirus is from cats and dogs.

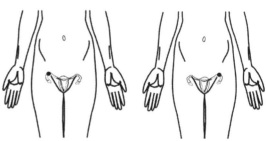

Main cause of infertility in women
(Sperm goes in, reaching tubal area
with the + charge of the parvovirus
and is rejected by charge)
Is in one of the tubes--check both.

FALLOPIAN TUBE/OVARY
Pair indicates ectopic pregnancy
Menstruation continues, as ovary
releases eggs (which should not be
the case in pregnancy). Fallopian
tube may begin to hurt.
If there is no pain, find which tube
contains the pregnancy. Goiz suggests

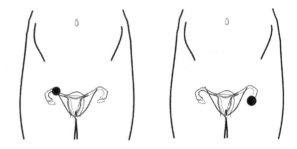

pushing the fertilized egg along the tube (with a magnet of same charge as the egg) and
into the uterus but to be done only in very early stages of pregnancy.

FEMUR
The thigh bone

FEMUR/FEMUR
Reservoir of mycosis (fungus)

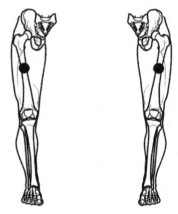

FLANK
At side of waist

FLANK/FLANK
Intestinal Yersinia pestis bacteria,
responsible for plague, transmitted by fleas. Check other areas
of *yersinia pestis*.

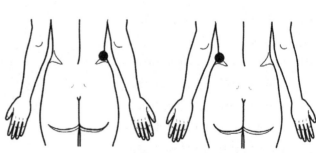

FOREHEAD
Above eyebrows

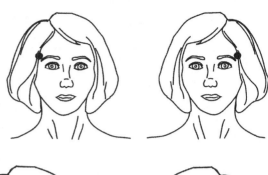

FOREHEAD SINUS/ FOREHEAD SINUS
On sides of forehead
Viral sinusitis

FRONTAL
FRONTAL/FRONTAL
Sinusitis virus

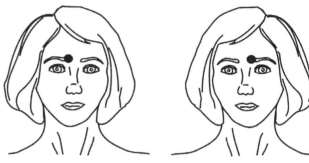

GALLBLADDER
On edge of rib, right side
(Under liver at bottom of men's
front pocket)

GALLBLADDER/GALLBLADDER
Special pair Prada
A reservoir of many viruses,
including Hepatitis B and
HIV 1, so after it is
impacted, the viruses go to
their "regular" places.

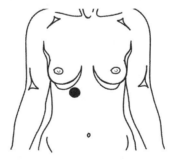
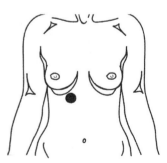

If the person's gallbladder has
been removed,
the energy stays in the stub
and can become polarized.

If this pair is detected, also depolarize
Pleura/Liver (Hepatitis B)
And Thymus/Rectum (HIV 1)

GALLBLADDER/RIGHT KIDNEY
Common cold virus
Make sure it is not an allergy

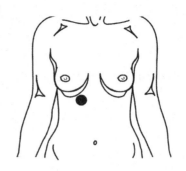 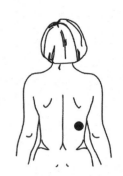

GALLBLADDER DUCT
To left of neck of gallbladder

GALLBLADDER DUCT/RIGHT KIDNEY
Spirochete bacteria
Cause of false diabetes,
Digestive problems

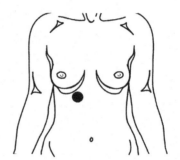 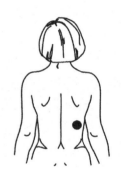

GLUTEUS
In seat—check various points,
going all around the area

GLUTEUS/GLUTEUS
Hookworm parasites or other
intestinal parasites

Can offer
potassium or epazote tea after
treatment with magnets

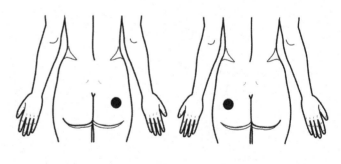

GLUTEUS/PYLORUS
Veillonela bacteria
Can cause root canal
infections,
nasal discharge

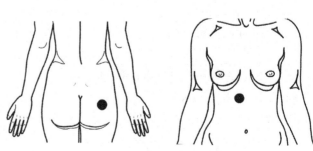

HAND
On palm of hand

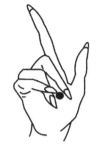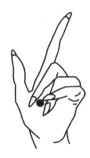

HAND/HAND
Plasmodium parasite
Transmitted by mosquito.

Causes malaria
Recurring fevers, chills,
acute digestive problems

HAND/BLADDER
Hand point on <u>back </u>of hand
Gives relief of pain on back of hand.

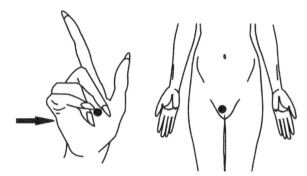

HEPATIC LIGAMENT
On liver above edge of ribs a little
Below breast on right

HEPATIC LIGAMENT/RIGHT KIDNEY
Adeno virus—hard to detect
Likes to pair up with parvovirus

Gives inflammation of lymphatics
(the ganglion)
fever, distention of abdomen,
false AIDS
respiratory diseases,
tumors.
Gives conjunctivitis, which should be treated with
both Hepatic Ligament/Right Kidney plus
Canthus/Canthus.

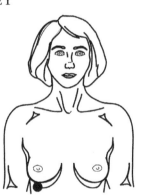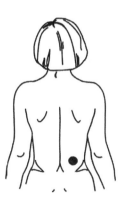

HEPATIC, RETRO/HEPATIC, RETRO

Below hepatic ligament on right side.
Toxocara parasite giving mange-like
symptoms

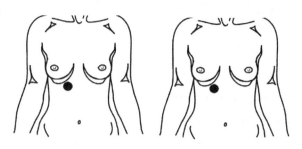

HIATUS

Under thymus at point where
Two ribs are apart

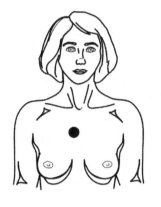
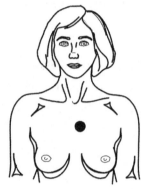

HIATUS/ESOPHAGUS

Enterobacter pneumonia bacteria
Pulmonary problems

HIATUS/RIGHT TESTICLE

Helicobacter pilori bacteria
At first, severe gastritis followed by
gastric ulcers,
Alters sperm production,
Bad digestion, Diaphragmatic hernia,
can give false diabetes

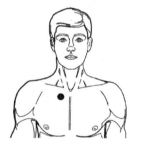
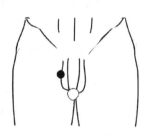

HIP

At hip bone

HIP/HIP

Chlamydia psittaci (*pneumonia*) bacteria

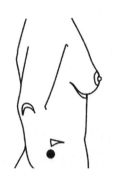
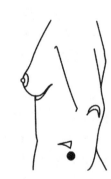

Affects coagulation systems and produces
bleeding, simulates pneumonia, In women it gives vaginal flux and bleeding.
Is main cause of cervical-uterine cancer

Nosebleed (epistaxis)
If associated with *Pseudomona* or *Yersinia*
gives false cancer,
problems in lungs, gives toxins
to the lungs, and if associated with
tuberculosis, there will be much
blood in lungs.

HUMERUS
Upper arm bone

HUMERUS/HUMERUS
Enterobacter pneumonia
Transmitted by dog and cat.
Respiratory problems
Lung disorders

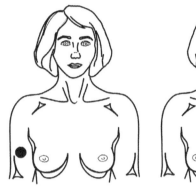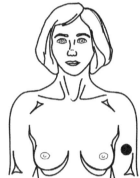

HYPOTHALAMUS
Deep within brain:
Put magnet on forehead
just above center point of pituitary gland

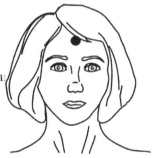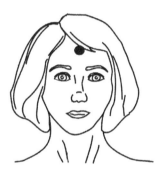

SPLEEN/HYPOTHALAMUS
Gives sluggishness
Is psycho-emotional point

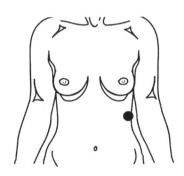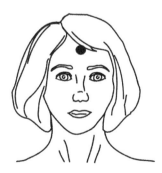

ILIAC

On iliac bone, bilateral
(Below waist on back of hip)

ILIAC/ILIAC
Special pair Elena
Dysfunctions of digestive tract
Sluggishness of intestines
Overweight from poor digestion of foods
Constipation
Need to do this pair two or three times

For varicose veins, do ILIAC/ILIAC and
Also rest feet up in air daily. Check
in pelvic area. Also, varicose ulcers are
From leprosy and came to Mexico from the
Chinese immigrants.

ILIAC CREST

ILIAC CREST/ILIAC CREST
On outer border of pelvic girdle

Trypanosoma gambiense bacteria giving
African sleeping sickness

ILEOCECAL VALVE

Between ileum termination and caecum
Where large intestine begins

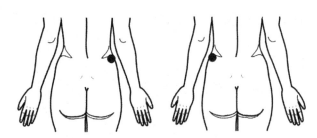

ILEOCECAL VALVE/RIGHT KIDNEY
Trichomonas micro organism
This is one point that is difficult
To scan for and find.
In women, can cause fallopian tube
infections, infection of covering of liver;
in men, pain in testis, narrowing of

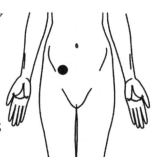
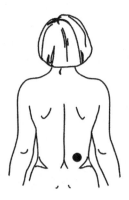

urethra; in women and men, can be
conjunctivitis ; in newborns, can be
conjunctivitis and pneumonia.
Treat both partners to avoid reinfection
Check also in Caecum/Caecum.

INDEX FINGER
Escherichia coli bacteria

INDEX FINGER/INDEX FINGER
For heightening immune system,
getting rid of fungus.
(Someone other than
Goiz found this BMP).

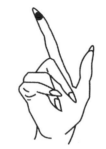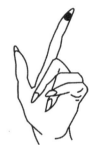

INGUINAL NERVE
Goes from top of femur to bladder
The point is on front of body at crease where
Legs hook on to trunk of body

INGUINAL NERVE/INGUINAL NERVE
HIV 3 virus (still under study)
Reservoir of viruses

Gives chronic diseases
Lower back pain

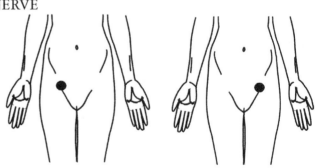

RIGHT INGUINAL NERVE (+ pole)/JOINTS (- pole)
Not a regular BMP
Gives articular rheumatism,
Isolated, noninfectious joint problems
For hip pain, try this: Put magnets on
pain and one on right inguinal nerve. Can
Also help for leg or arm pain

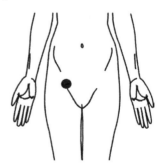

Check
Joints
In
body

INGUINAL NERVE/LIVER

Roseola virus—Common in children under 3.

Viral infection from Herpes 6 virus.

Flat eruptions on chest, back, arms

Inflammation of neck ganglion

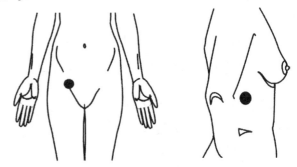

INTERCILIAR

Between eyebrows

INTERCILIAR/RACHIDIAN BULB

Special BMP David

Defines and affects character.

Provokes personality changes.

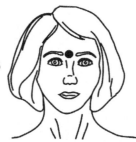
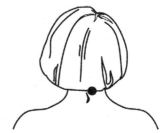

INTERCILIAR/SACRUM

Reservoir for parasites

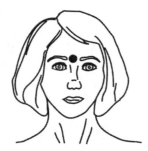
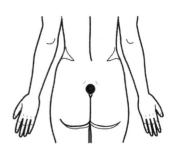

INTER ILIAC

Below waist on back of hip

INTERILIAC/SACRUM

This pair is a reservoir of parasites.

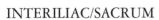
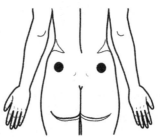
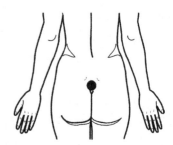

ISCHIUM

Posterior in bend of buttocks
on edge of pelvis

ISCHIUM/ISCHIUM

Onchocercosis parasite, which
are worms that multiply rapidly in a
patient's body, characterized by
nodules or bumps under the skin, an itching rash, eye tumors and loss of skin color and
possible elephantitis. Spread by bite of black fly, *onchocera volvulus*

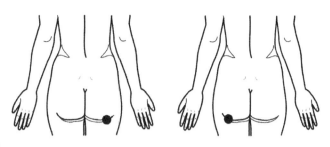

ISCHIUM BRANCH

Inner part of ischium

ISCHIUM BRANCH/ISCHIUM
BRANCH

Streptococcus C

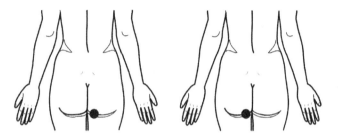

JOINTS

Articulations of body

JOINT/ KIDNEY OF SAME SIDE

Swelling from physical trauma
See also Inguinal nerve

Check
Joints
In
body

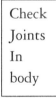
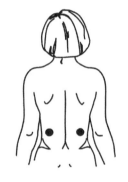

JUGULAR

Along jugular

JUGULAR/JUGULAR

Not regular BMP
Hypertension
Tetanus
Edema, mental confusion,
Fever, acute catarrh

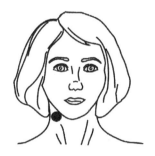
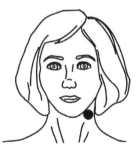

KIDNEY

In a crisis or after trauma, put magnets on the two kidneys.
Helpful for scorpion bites (poison similar to that of *Pneumococcus* an
Also, to help kidneys get rid of intoxications and infections,
put + magnet on kidney, - magnet on parietal.

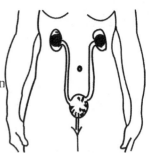

KIDNEY/KIDNEY
Clostridium tetani bacteria
(There are 4 kinds of Clostridium)
Some patients have had surgery
for this but condition
continues. Tetanus is toxic because of
metabolites expelled from kidney
which can hit the brain, causing
death.
Can exist in stump
of kidney. Often is cause of nephritis
and lowering of renal function.
Some patients have raised cretenin
levels (produced by liver)
and doctors think it is due to a
weakened kidney, but it isn't.
Edema, mental confusion,
fever, acute catarrh can
all result

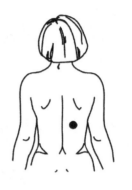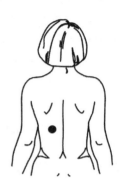

KIDNEY/OPPOSITE SACRUM
Intestinal dysfunction
Intestinal noises, gas, flatulence

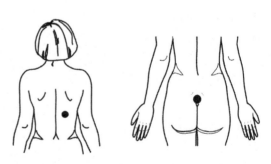

KIDNEY/OPPOSITE PARIETAL

Special pair Goiz

First special pair discovered and is only organ found so far that can cause a shortening of the leg of the polarized side of the body.

Can affect central nervous system. and symptomology can cross over to other side of body, giving motor and subtle disturbances of conduct.

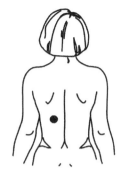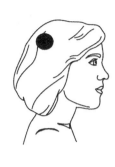

KIDNEY/CHEEKBONE

Malaria

Produces rheumatic complications, tiredness, pain, fibromyalgia

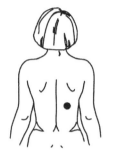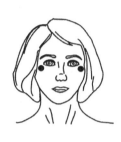

KIDNEY/RENAL CAPSULE

Special pair Ale

Reservoir for HIV and perhaps other viruses. When this pair is depolarized bacteria and viruses immediately go to Thymus/Rectum.

This is a vertical pair and can be on right or left side, with both on same side. Change toothbrushes when viruses are present.

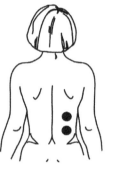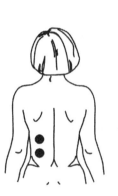

KIDNEY/URETER

Both magnets on same side

Special pair Machin

Nephritic stones or colic

In women, menstrual pain

Use this for pain if passing a kidney stone

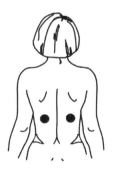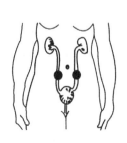

RIGHT KIDNEY/DUODENUM
Diabetes mellitus
This is not a regular pair. It is a special pair.
If one's urine is very alkaline, it is not
diabetes. Is diabetes only when it becomes
very acid and the insulin production of the
pancreas is affected.

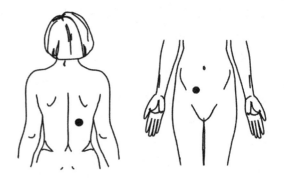

RIGHT KIDNEY/LIVER
Morganella typhus
Gives hepatic cirrhosis (though 80%,
according to Goiz, are not true hepatic
cirrhosis) With Morganella, it is the
Morganella giving off the pus, not liver

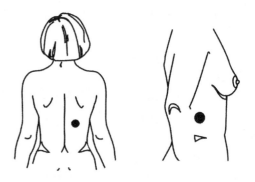

KNEE LIGAMENT
Inner side of knee

KNEE LIGAMENT / MALLEOLUS
Micro sporum fungus

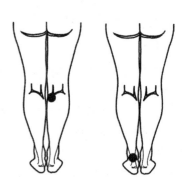

LACHRYMAL
Almost at corner of eye where tears come

LACHRYMAL/LACHRYMAL
Klebsiella pneumonia bacteria
Rhinitis, laryngitis
Cough, nosebleed.
(Others giving nosebleed:
Dengue, *anthrax*, Cytomegalovirus,
and Haemophilus influenza)

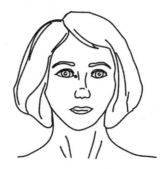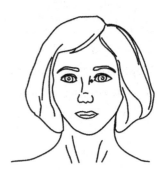

LARYNX

Above thyroid at
Middle of neck
Put magnets one over the
other a little above thyroid

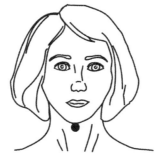
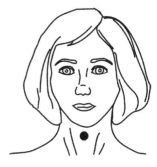

LARYNX/LARYNX

Bordetella pertussis bacteria
Whooping cough
Chronic cough
These bacteria are mostly from
milk products or are spread from person to person.

LATISSIMUS DORSI

A pair of large, triangular
muscles of back
extending from under scapula to waist
Can be any place along muscle

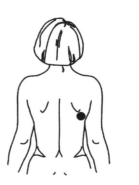
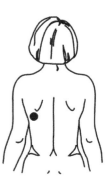

LATISSIMUS DORSI/LATISSIMUS DORSI

Yersinia pestis –goes to lungs and is
very problematic.
Gives pneumonia.

LIGAMENT

A little below bottom
right gall bladder, front and straight
through to back side

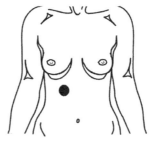
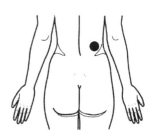

LIGAMENT/RIGHT KIDNEY

Adeno virus
This virus causes problems with
upper lung infection or stomach
and intestinal infection.

LIVER
Large, under pleura; try several points
to locate point of greater polarization.

LIVER/LIVER
Hepatitis C (toxin)
Is toxic, neither virus nor bacteria, acquired
from eating yellow fats and raw oils
(such as margarine) or from many
allopathic medicines.
Put magnets one above another at about
arm bend level
Liver/Liver can also be involved with vision problems.

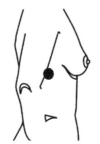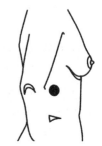

LIVER/LEFT KIDNEY
Posterior lobe of liver
Hepatic amoeba parasite
Occurs when the amoeba goes from pylorus to
liver, causing abscess.
Is hepatic amoebeasis, which is common.

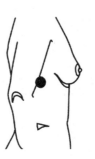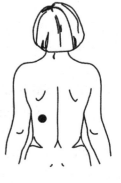

LIVER/PLEURA
Viral hepatitis

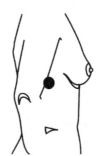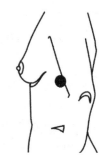

LIVER/PYLORUS
Pinworm parasite

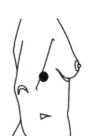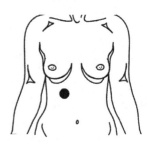

LIVER/RIGHT KIDNEY

Enlarged or too fatty liver
In cases of cirrhosis, ask body what % of
liver is destroyed. According to Goiz,
this organ can easily regenerate.

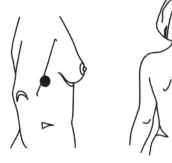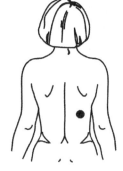

LIVER/SPLEEN

Brucella bacteria
Brucellosis

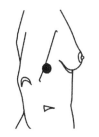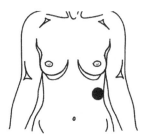

LUMBAR

Waist area on spine

4TH LUMBAR/4TH LUMBAR

Neisseria gonorrhea bacteria

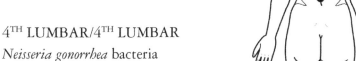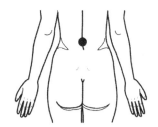

LUMBAR PLEXUS

On 4th lumbar at waist
LUMBAR PLEXUS/LUMBAR PLEXUS
Enterococcus bacteria
Gives digestion problem

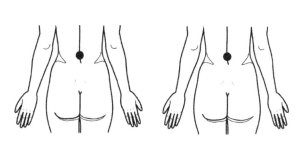

MALAR

Cheek

MALAR/MALAR

Enterovirus
Very aggressive

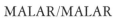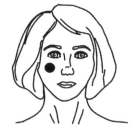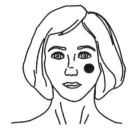

Headache, dizziness diarrhea,
Is confused with HIV
to give false AIDS

MALAR/STERNUM
Enterovirus
(which flourishes mostly in the
intestinal tract)

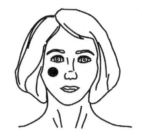 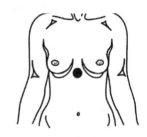

MALLEOLUS
Ankle

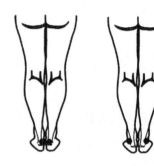

MALLEOLUS/MALLEOLUS
Indicates fungus
With both magnets on inside of
ankle, or both on outside of
ankle

MANDIBLE
Various points on jawbone from chin to angle

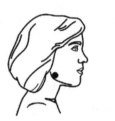 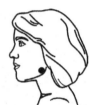

MANDIBLE/MANDIBLE
Neisseria gonorrhea bacteria

Gingivitis,
Gonorrhea
Facial paralysis
If this condition is serious, put a negative magnet
under the chin and two positive magnets on each side
along mandible.

Arthritis is caused by this.
Rheumatism is caused by a combination of the
gonococcal and meningococcal micro organisms
Is from urethral or sexual transmission.

MANGO

Under location where the clavicle bones join together

MANGO/MANGO
Coxsackievirus

One of the 30 viruses that
Infect the intestines.

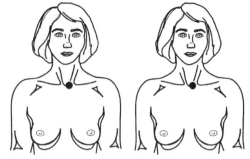

MASTOID

Small bone behind ear

MASTOID/MASTOID
Filaria parasite which makes
a toxin that travels to the
brain and creates epilepsy
and seizures.
Dizziness.
Results in alterations through
intracranial tumors.
Carried by fly

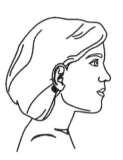
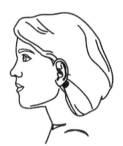

MAXILLARY SINUS

A hole in upper jaw next to nasal cavity

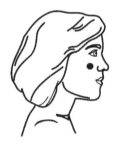
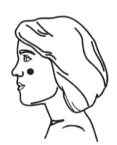

MAXILLARY SINUS/MAXILLARY SINUS
Gives viral sinusitis

MEDIASTINUM

Under thymus and affects thymus. In a portion of the
space in middle of chest, between sacs containing lungs.
It extends from breastbone (sternum) to spine. It contains all
of chest organs except lungs.

INFERIOR MEDIASTINUM/
SUPERIOR MEDIASTINUM

Proteus mirabilis

Is main cause of immune deficiency
as it affects thymus.
Use to heighten a lowered immune system.
Dysfunction of thymus
Inflammation of mediastinum
(= mediastinitis, with laryngeal,
pulmonary and bronchial symptoms)
Gives false AIDS if combined with another virus.
It traps the thymus anatomically as well
as functionally.

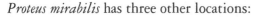

Proteus mirabilis has three other locations:
1) Costal/Costal, which gives pleuritis
and causes bleeding
2) Sacrum/Sacrum, gives infertility,
muscle problems.
3) Renal capsule/Renal capsule Gives lupus.

MOLE

Any mole on any part of body

MOLE/KIDNEY SAME SIDE
Hanta virus
Make sure to check all moles.

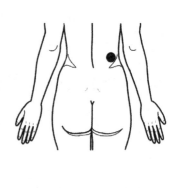

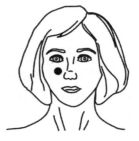

NASAL SINUS

On cheek bone, below eye,
between nose and cheek

NASAL SINUS/NASAL SINUS
Viral sinusitis virus

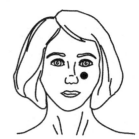

NECK

Above the scapula on back by neck
But not on neck

NECK/NECK
Blastocystis hominis fungus

Goes to lung and radiates to
skin, bladder and prostate

NECK/FEMUR
To kill fungus

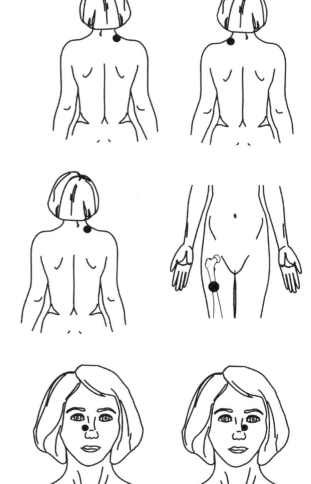

NOSE

Inferior part of nose

NOSE/NOSE
Toxoides--not bacterium or virus
Product of allergies in nose
Do here for vision problems

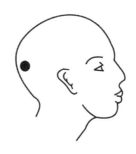

OCCIPITAL

Behind mastoid

OCCIPITAL/OCCIPITAL
Epstein-Barr virus

Dizziness, irritability,
Mental confusion, Neurological symptoms,
Fatigue
Causes a change in behavior and in
equilibrium (as does Pole/Pole)

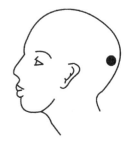

ORBITAL FLOOR

Point at outer lower corner of eye

ORBITAL FLOOR/ORBITAL FLOOR
For Orf virus (gotten from sheep
Resulting in skin disease with blisters)

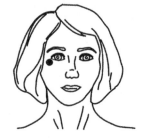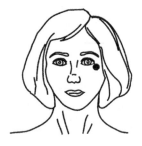

OVARY

Bilateral on sides of uterus

OVARY/OVARY
Ovarian dysfunction
Causes infertility

It is secondary to an inflammatory process.

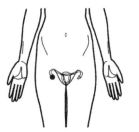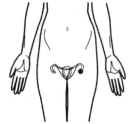

PANCREAS

Under and left of stomach above
navel

PANCREAS/PANCREAS
Special pair Ramses
At middle of pancreas and at
pancreas tail
Is there bad digestion?
Put two magnets on pancreas.
Working here can stop convulsions.
Heavy metal toxicity
can give deep psychological problems.
Makes people feel like they need sleep
as it affects potassium metabolism.
Can be from toxic seafood, excessive protein
Poisoning.

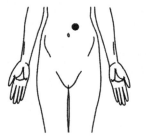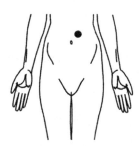

PANCREAS HEAD/ADRENALS

Above navel

Staphylococcus aureus cuag + and

Staphylococcus epidermis

Halitosis

Main cause of gastric reflux

Can cause cancer of pancreas head.

Can give false diabetes.

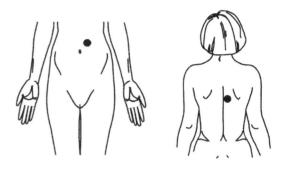

PANCREAS BODY/ PANCREAS TAIL

Special pair Ramses

Pancreatitis

Produces a toxin that generates a psychotic state in patient, with atypical conduct affecting the CNS (central nervous system).

Associated with Fasciola hepatica.

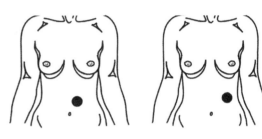

PANCREAS TAIL/LIVER

Clostridium botulinum bacteria

Botulism

Obtained from pickled, canned, bottled foods milk products; gives intestinal problems, muscular pain, colic and gas

(All Clostridium are involved in metastasis, according to Goiz)

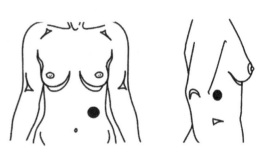

PANCREAS TIP/SPLEEN

Common wart

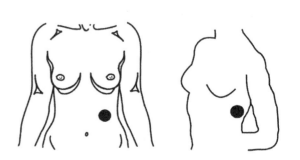

PANCREAS DUCT

Directly above bellybutton at waist

PANCREAS DUCT/LEFT KIDNEY

Spirochete bacteria
Causes false diabetes

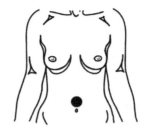
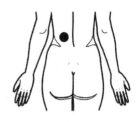

PARATHYROID

Under ear at thyroid height

PARATHYROID/PARATHYROID

Glandular dysfunction
Parathyroid fails from stress
Parathyroid secretes calcitonin, which gives
calcium to bones and regulates calcium.

Gives syndrome of hypocalcemia, and leads to
osteoporosis.
This pair can help osteoporosis, even in menopause.

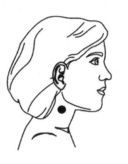
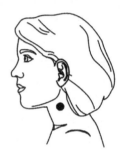

PARIETAL

Over parietal bone

PARIETAL/PARIETAL

Viral encephalitis virus
This virus usually transferred from
animals to humans, but not usually
from humans to animals.
(Parietal/Parietal
can alleviate distemper in puppies).
Can affect vision. giving blindness, cataracts.
sleeping sickness or cerebral fever,
confusion, mucus and tear secretion.

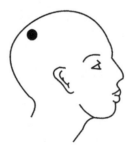
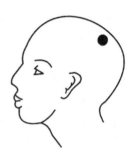

Good for helping to treat rattlesnake bite.

PARIETAL/LEFT KIDNEY
Plasmodium vivax protozoa (from
mosquito) giving
common tertian malaria

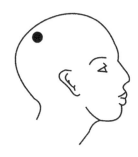
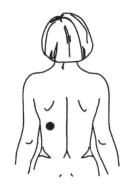

PARIETAL/OPPOSITE KIDNEY
Special pair Goiz (positive
polarization of kidney of same side as
short leg).
Check polarities as the person now has
one half of the body shorter than the
other and it should be corrected before
proceeding with scanning.
Causes renal, cerebral, or pulmonary problems.
Found in most bronchitis cases.
It gives "heavy head" with deafness and Tiredness.
Special pair Goiz can also be located in ear or parotid and opposite kidney.

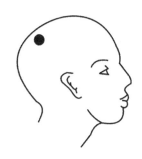
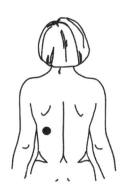

PARIETAL/ TRANSVERSE COLON
Entamoeba histolytic parasite. Can
be parietal on both sides at same time.
Transverse colon point is under bellybutton
Gives cerebral cysts
Can cause pain, insomnia, other
mental or neurological problems.

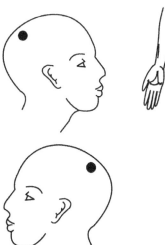
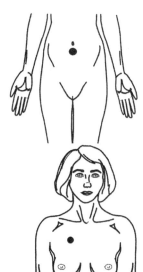

LEFT PARIETAL/THYMUS
Rubeola

PAROTID

Below jawbone under and in front of ear

PAROTID/PAROTID

Special pair Lolita
The parotid gland has a
direct influence on the hormone
production of the parathyroid,
the thyroid, and the pancreas through
its secretion of parotina.
Parotina leads to production of thyroxin,

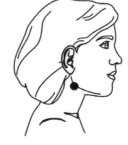
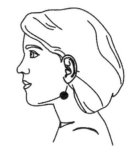

insulin, and calcitonin which in turn, can affect digestion and body weight
disturbances and calcium absorption and bone density. Parotid dysfunction causes
a lowering of hormones.

Goiz says if you find Parotid/Parotid, also check the person
for presence of Pudendal/Pudendal. With Parotid/Parotid
plus Pudendal/Pudendal, it is parotiditis, which indicates
parotiditis virus. Parotiditis in a male
can cause infertility

PELVIS

CLITORIS/PELVIS
Spirochete E.

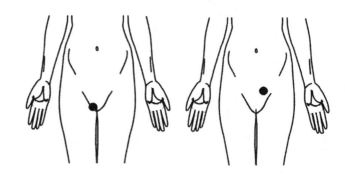

PENIS

Anterior at joining of legs to
trunk of body

PENIS/THYMUS
Erectile dysfunction

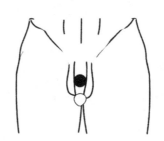
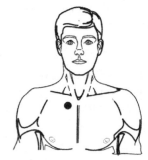

PERICARDIUM
A little to left of cardia enclosing heart

PERICARDIUM/PERICARDIUM
Staphylococcus aureus coag+ bacteria

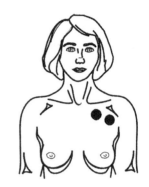

This was spread by hospital air conditioners
Can be lethal if it is on both sides, according to
Goiz.
Gives Pericarditis,
heart arrythmia and cardiac pathology

PERIHEPATIC
On edge of ribs by liver
Put magnets horizontally

PERIHEPATIC/PERIHEPATIC
Morganella typhus bacteria,
very aggressive bacteria.

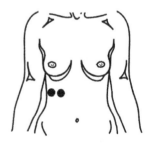

Is from bad meat, poorly cooked meat
Causes problems with liver,
anorexia, severe digestive problems,
diarrhea, fever
Is confused with cirrhosis of liver
Vegetarians who do not eat meat
can get it if they eat vegetables
refrigerated next to bad meat—common
in some restaurants.

This appears on edge of liver, and when
doctors do a biopsy of the liver,
they can contaminate the sample and
call it cirrhosis of the liver.

PERIRENAL
Surrounding the kidney

PERIRENAL/PERI RENAL
Bovine tuberculosis.

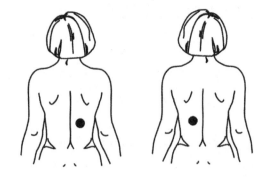

PERITONEUM
Lining of abdominal cavity

PERITONEUM/PLEURA
Moises special pair
Reservoir of bacteria
Fairly rare
Depolarize it with TWO pairs
of magnets simultaneously, one pair
on each side of body, placing
lower magnets over intestinal walls on
front part of body; upper magnets
over pleura under armpits.

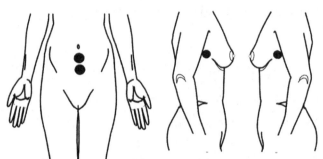

PINEAL
Highest point of cranium

PINEAL/PINEAL (horizontal)
Pineal dysfunction
Vitiligio or hypochromia
Acts on pigments, sexuality
and adrenals.
Is damaged by trauma

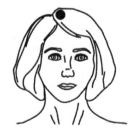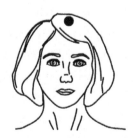

PINEAL/RACHIDIAN BULB
Guillan barre virus
or polyradiculo neuritis, which can give
ventilation paralysis
Paralysis and weakness of members
Dizziness, fatigue
Very contagious.

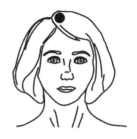 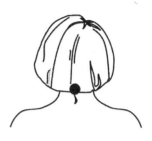

Goiz tells us this pair is the most common cause of quadriplegia.
It causes death due to the paralysis of the diaphragm and death
results from not breathing.

PITUITARY
In center of forehead

PITUITARY/PITUITARY
Glandular dysfunction
Galactorrhea (Milk flow not related to
childbirth or nursing—may be a symptom of
pituitary gland tumor)

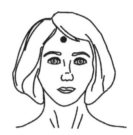 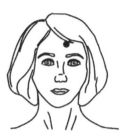

PITUITARY/BLADDER
Common dengue virus
(as opposed to Rachidian bulb /Bladder,
hemorrhagic type dengue)
From mosquito bites
Joint pains,
Like cold with mucus
Lowers interferon level

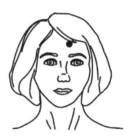 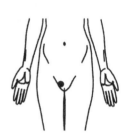

PITUITARY/ RACHIDIAN BULB
Diabetes insipid—not a regular
biomagnetic pair
as it lacks virus-bacteria presence
Sickness of metabolism and of thirst
Most patients can be cured of this.

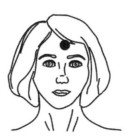 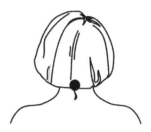

PITUITARY/RIGHT OVARY

Special pair Carmen
Involved with amenorrhea (suppression
or absence of menstruation) and
dysmenorrha (difficult or painful
menstruation) or dysfunction of ovaries

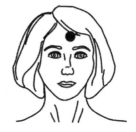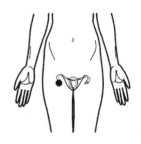

PLANTAR ARCH

Of sole of foot

PLANTAR ARCH/PLANTAR ARCH

Paramoxivirus, a member of a family of
viruses that includes those causing mumps and
certain lung infections. Also Ebola.

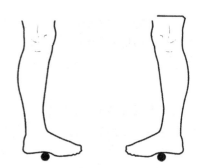

PLEURA

Lining of thoracic cavity
Scan under armpits but at
mid-liver level.

PLEURA/PLEURA: 1 side

Pseudomona aeruginosa bacteria
Both magnets impact on same side,
Right or left

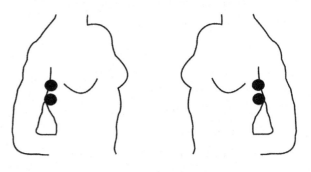

PLEURA/PLEURA: 2 sides

Pleuritis virus
One magnet on
left side, one on right side.
Gives pleuritis
Is rare, but simulates pneumonia
or bronchitis with fever

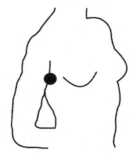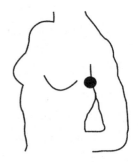

RIGHT PLEURA/ LIVER
Hepatitis B (DNA virus)
This gives fatigue and colitis.
Is curable with magnets.

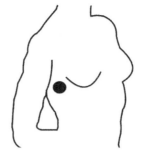 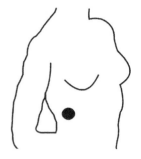

POLE
At "horns"

POLE/POLE
Special pair Abraham
Dyslexia treatable here
Can control bulimia. Connected with false
pregnancy. This corrects vertical equilibrium.
(For horizontal equilibrium, do Ear/Ear)

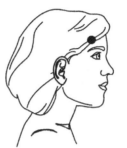 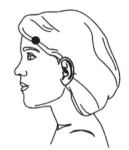

POLYGON
Over ear next to temple

POLYGON/POLYGON
Reovirus
Problems of breathing and in
digestive tract

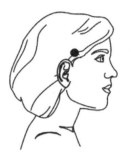 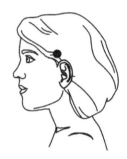

POPLITEAL
At knee bend, posterior

POPLITEAL/POPLITEAL
Pneumococcus or Pneumonia bacteria
Causes congestion in pelvis or lungs.
Goes from pelvic cavity to lungs
giving pneumonia
Look for this in women with pelvic infection.

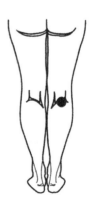 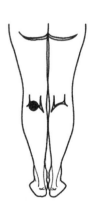

Pneumococcus gives explosive congestions.

PROSTATE

Surrounding urethra at bladder--located
between testicles

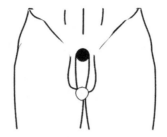 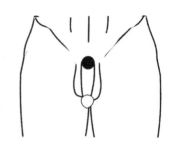

PROSTATE/PROSTATE

Glandular dysfunction

PROSTATE/RECTUM

Papiloma virus

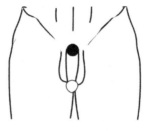 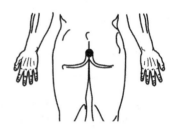

Often in cases of papiloma virus,
doctors call it cancer or pre cancer.
Is confused with Parvo virus, corona
virus and other viruses in that area.
Can give vaginal warts in women.
If it associates with leprosy,
it produces a myoma (tumor of muscle tissue) or cyst.

If Prostate/Rectum is in a male, check him for energy problems
in areas corresponding to ovaries, fallopian tubes, uterus.
If Prostate/Rectum is in a female, check her for energy
problems in areas corresponding to prostate and testicles.

Can be confused with Parvo virus.

PUDENDAL

Line or crease between trunk of body and legs

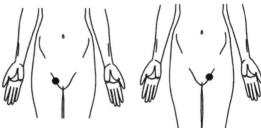

PUDENDAL/PUDENDAL

Parotiditis virus
Gives mumps. Affects the testicles and bladder.
If Pudendal/Pudendal is present, check also
for Parotid/Parotid. Together, Pudendal/
Pudendal + Parotid/Parotid = Parotiditis.
Parotiditis can produce infertility in male.
Any problems in this area can be caused by parotiditis

PYLORUS

Under gallbladder in front of lower central part of liver (to right of central line from chin to navel)

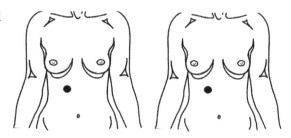

PYLORUS/PYLORUS
Medication intoxication

PYLORUS/LEFT KIDNEY
Intestinal amoebeasis parasite.
Very toxic. Gives vomit or metal taste in mouth
(When amoebeasis parasite goes to liver, it is hepatic amoebeasis, which is often wrongly called hepatitis. It can also go to thorax and bronchials)

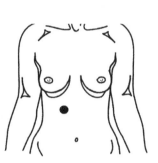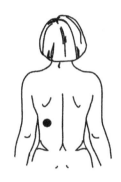

PYLORUS/LIVER
Pinworm parasite (*Enterobius vermicularis*)
Can give Hepatitis J
Severe liver problems
Gives digestive problems
Worms can give false diabetes
Liver placement: on front

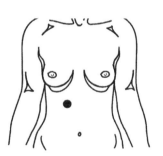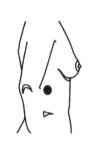

PYLORUS/OPPOSITE KIDNEY
Causes hot flashes and flushing or reddening of neck and facial skin

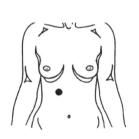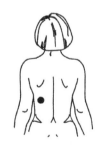

PYLORUS/URETER
Intestinal mycelia (a mass of threadlike strands found on most fungi. Also called hypha).

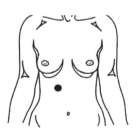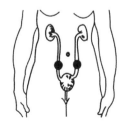

QUADRATE

On back above waist on lumbar region
Holds up last rib on each side of spine

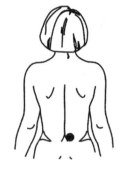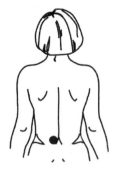

QUADRATE/QUADRATE

Syphilis bacillus

(See also Deltoid, Middle)

QUADRICEPS

Anterior part of thighs; need to check
along entire length from top of
upper leg to down above knee

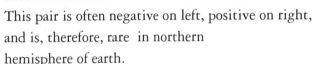

QUADRICEPS/QUADRICEPS

Special pair Magda
A phenomenon from insecticides, toxins
or from bismuth intoxication
causing waist and hip pain,
false rheumatism.
This pair is often negative on left, positive on right,
and is, therefore, rare in northern
hemisphere of earth.
Bismuth can intoxicate. Bismuth is used
on plants and parasites. Sometimes, in eating plants,
we get too much bismuth—especially
vegetarians. Try this pair for diabetes.

RACHIDIAN BULB

At nape of neck straight over from ear

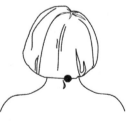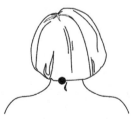

RACHIDIAN BULB/RACHIDIAN BULB
Insomnia

RACHIDIAN BULB/BLADDER

Hemorrhagic dengue virus
Secretes large quantities of mucoproteins
Can cause death.
Upon impacting the pair,
vomiting is likely
Impact this pair for incontinence.
Incontinence from an inflammation of the
nerves so usually the positive magnet is on
bladder.

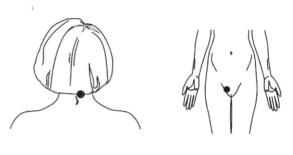

RACHIDIAN BULB/CEREBELLUM

Newcastle virus
From eating improperly cooked chicken (if
it still has any red in it).
Causes dizziness, uneven and staggering walk,
equilibrium of position problems,
aggressive behavior, fatigue,
mental retardation.

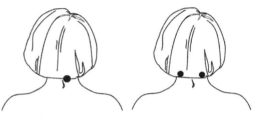

Muscular coordination of thorax, and
regulation of affected inspiration-expiration.
Produces cerebral ataxia which can cause death.

This pair is one of three to check for equilibrium
and dizziness. The other two are:
1)Middle Ear/Middle Ear (vertical equilibrium)
2) Pole/Pole (horizontal equilibrium)

RACHIDIAN BULB/THYROID

Meningitis virus
Is a DNA pathogen
Affects nervous system
Inflammation of meninges

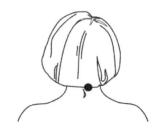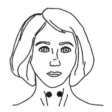

191

RADIUS

Anterior, shorter, thicker bone of forearm on Thumb side

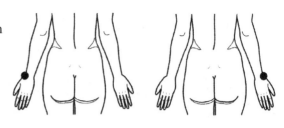

RADIUS/RADIUS
Microsporum fungus

RECTUM

Below coccyx

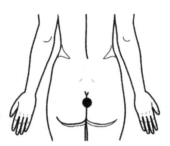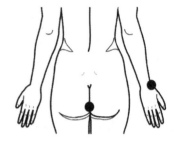

RECTUM/RECTUM
Pseudomona aeruginosa bacteria
(At times this bacterium goes to Pleura/Pleura, but then it is with both points on same side of body)
Believed to originate metastasis in cancer
Put one magnet on rectum, another above rectum.

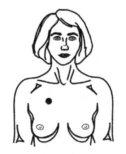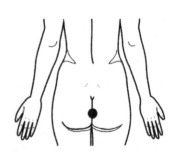

THYMUS/RECTUM
AIDS HIV
The virus is in rectum

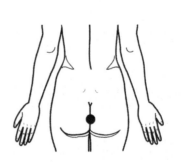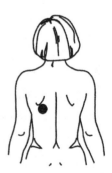

RECTUM/ADRENAL
Leptospira parasite
Gives effects similar to those of mange.
Transmitted by animals.

RENAL CAPSULE

Goes from kidney almost to scapula
Can be extensive, but if it is only at one
point, that would be at the kidney.

RENAL CAPSULE/RENAL CAPSULE

Proteus mirabilis bacteria
Produces true systemic lupus
This can cause infertility, too, as
uterus is blocked.

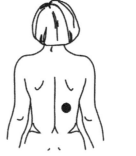 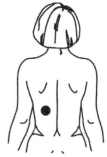

If someone has been diagnosed with lupus
and it is not in the renal capsule, it
probably is false lupus.
("lupus" = "lobo" = wolf face with stains)

RIB

Below clavicle

RIB/RIB

Onychomycosis (any fungal infection
of the nails)

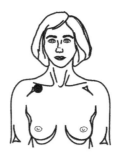 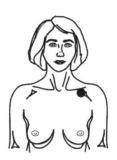

RIB #1/ RIB #1

Trycophyte fungus
Infects skin, hair and nails.

ROTULA

Round bone on front of knee

ROTULA/ROTULA

Gives fear
(as in "My knees were shaking.")

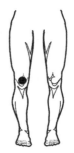 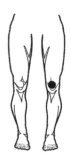

SACRUM
Above coccyx

SACRUM/SACRUM
Proteus mirabilis bacteria
Produces irritation, infection and
degeneration of end of tailbone
Infertility, muscular problems
in movement and joints of
lower members

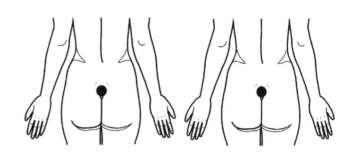

SACRUM/FEMUR
Norwalk virus, which gives up to
50% of gastroenteritis problems in
world—nausea, vomiting, diarrhea,
abdominal pain
Also food poisoning: in U.S. often
linked to eating raw oysters.

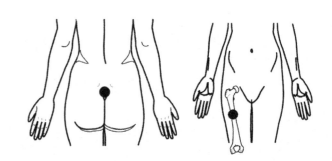

SCAPULA
Shoulder blade

SCAPULA/SCAPULA
Mycobacterium lepra bacteria
Leprosy
Malignancy factor in cancer
Is very aggressive, cause of true cancer
Produces toxins such as
lysozyme, goes to skin and
destroys it, produces *dedos de tambor*
(fat or inflamed fingers).
Goiz says 30% of Mexicans have this.
Gives bronchitis and in advanced cases,
gives skin problems resembling skin
coming off after sunburn.
If associated with a virus, can cause
a cataract.

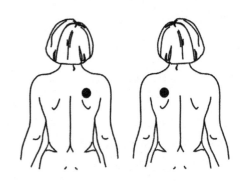

The *Mycobacterium lepra* can produce:

1) if it goes to the kidney: calcium deposits (kidney stones)

2) if it goes to the lung: emphysema

3) if it goes to the eyes: varicose ulcers, cataracts

Goiz says impacting a kidney stone with a magnet
will not break it up, as it is an inert substance and won't react to the
magnetic energy. Some of his students have been able to break up kidney stones with this pair.

SCIATIC
Various points between knee and
buttocks, posterior

SCIATIC/SCIATIC
Poliomyelitis virus
Pain in legs, muscular insufficiency
Low back pain, nervous system alterations
Paralysis and muscular dyskinesia (impaired ability
to make voluntary movements)
Goiz says the act of forgiveness
or pardoning (if the person carries a grudge)
can help relieve this BMP.

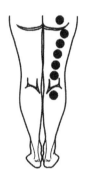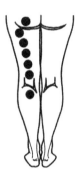

Often, due to polio vaccination when the
polio energy continues living in the body.

SINOATRIAL-ATRIOVENTRICULAR
Node of heart

SINOATRIAL-ATRIOVENTRICULAR /
LEFT KIDNEY

This is a special pair (termed Ana Alicia by
Goiz)
For tachycardia (excessive velocity of
Heart beat rhythm)

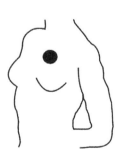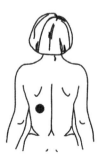

SPLEEN
Above pancreas tail at
ribs 11 and 12.

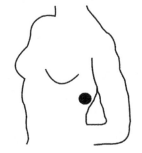 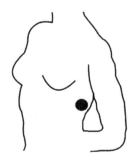

SPLEEN/SPLEEN
Yersinia pestis bacteria
or spleen dysfunction
Bronchitis type laryngeal cough
Vaginal flux in women
Azoospermia in men
Put the magnets side by side horizontally

SPLEEN/DUODENUM
Leukemia.

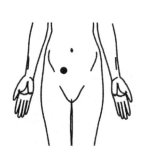

Not a regular pair but a pathology.
If spleen is affected, it affects the blood.
Whatever pathology affects the spleen can
give leukemia-type symptoms.
(Goiz says 90% of "leukemia" is false. There is only
a change in white blood cell quantity, not in the genetics.
They call it cancer, but the cells are not abnormal
And cancer implies a change in the cells! The
spleen is swollen and producing many cells,
but not abnormal ones, according to Goiz.)
Is confused with brucellosis;
Gives pulmonary problems

SPLEEN/HYPOTHALAMUS
Psycho instinctive pair relating
to sluggishness

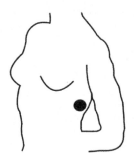 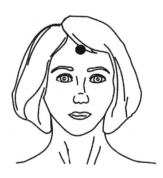

SPLEEN/LIVER

Brucellosis bacteria
or Maltese fever
From eating infected yogurt and cream, source
of "90%" of false leukemia.
Is confused with leukemia, giving
false leukemia; with respiratory and
pulmonary problems such as
bronchitis.
Put magnets at same level on sides of chest,
above tail of pancreas and on liver

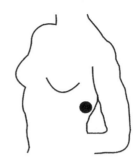
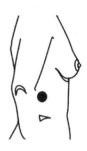

SPLEEN/PANCREAS
For common wart virus

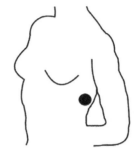
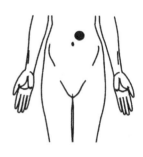

STERNOCLEIDOMASTOID
(SCM)
Under mastoid under ears

SCM/SCM
Sympathetic nerve system dysfunction
Alterations in sympathetic nerve
system such as poor circulation,
sweating, palpitation,
irritable colon
Goiz asks: Why do so many
women have headaches? Because
their sexual organs irritate parasympathetic
nerves, causing headaches.
Can often cure them in SCM/SCM or in pelvis
or with descending colon.

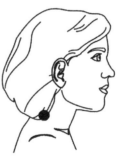
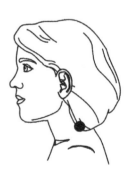

STERNUM
At base of sternum

STERNUM/ADRENALS
Is a special BMP called Lucio.
Regulates number of red blood
cells in blood (hemotochryte)

Use for anemia.
For polyglobulina (excess of red blood cells)

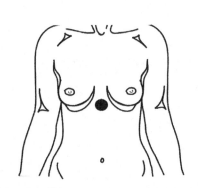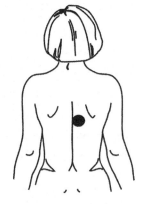

STERNUM/LIVER
Hemorrhagic conjunctiva (bleeding of
the conjunctiva, the mucous membrane
lining inner surface of eyelid and
exposed surface of eyeball), bruises,
bloody discharges

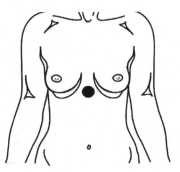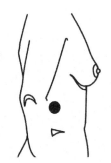

STOMACH
Under cardia a little to left

STOMACH/STOMACH
Stomach dysfunction
Stomach colic, bad digestion,
belching

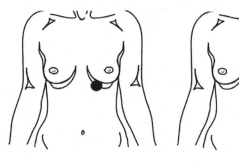

STOMACH/ADRENALS
Measles virus
Main cause of gastritis
(together with *helicobacter
pilori*) One woman got measles
from eating infected eggs.

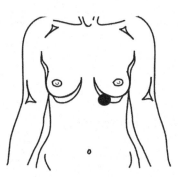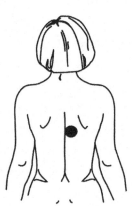

In a child is rather light, but in an
adult it always manifests with
high alimentary canal bleeding
and can give ulcers.

STOMACH/PYLORUS
Clostridium perfringens bacteria
Very aggressive
Gives digestive problems,
uterine infections
Can be from milk products

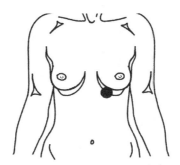 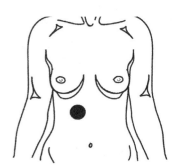

STUB/STUB
Special pair Guadalupe

Any stub or stump remaining from
an amputated organ or appendage.
can harbor and be a reservoir for
bacteria, viruses, parasites, or fungi.

(Case Specific)

SUBCLAVIAN
Under clavicle

SUBCLAVIAN/SUBCLAVIAN
Diphtheria bacillus
Trachea-bronchial problems (classified
by allopathic medicine as "asthma"),
chronic cough, diarrhea,
Main cause of general edema
Gives lung problems and allergies
Transmitted by milk products
Main cause of Hodgkin's (cancer
of the neck)
Makes liver extend
After impacting, there is much urine.

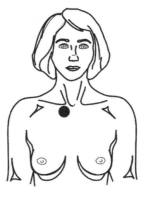 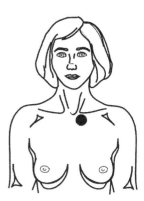

SUB DIAPHRAGM
Below diaphragm

SUB DIAPHRAGM/
SUB DIAPHRAGM
Cysticercosis, from poorly
cooked pork. Cysticercus,
the larval stage of pork

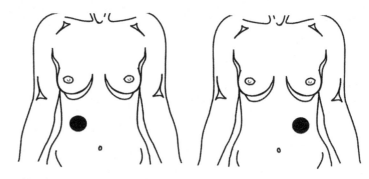

tapeworm infects the brain, muscles, and internal organs causing cysts, and if in brain,
headaches and even seizures.

SUPRACILIAR
Just above interciliar

SUPRACILIAR/RACHIDIAN BULB
Special pair Vivian
Alterations of anatomical
integrity. Sadness/depression
from losses (lacking an
appendage) or an abortion or
an unwanted pregnancy.
If an organ has been removed
in surgery, or a leg lost to
amputation this pair can help

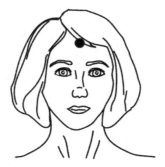
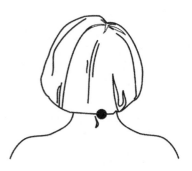

cancel the negative feeling from loss, whether physical or psychological. Also formed
upon losing a family member and feeling great loss. This point has also helped correct
over activity in children. Good for under activity, too, as in under activity of growth
process in dwarfs or children who have not developed. Use this to normalize growth.

SUPRA HEPATIC
Above liver

SUPRA HEPATIC/SUPRA HEPATIC
Clostridium malignum bacteria
(*Clostridium* is a genus of bacteria
that forms spores and needs no oxygen
to live.)

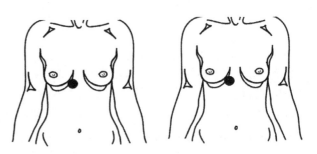

SUPRA PUBIC

Above pubis

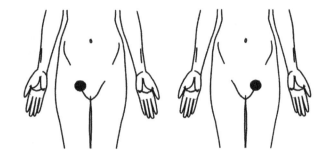

SUPRA PUBIC/ SUPRA PUBIC
HTLV virus
Magnets placed side by side.

SUPRASPINAL

On trapezium at side of neck, two
or three fingers away from neck

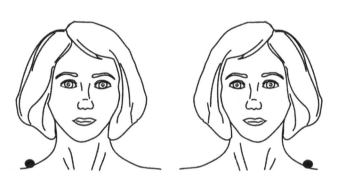

SUPRASPINAL/SUPRASPINAL
Mycobacterium tuberculosis
It gives abscesses in body
Can affect gall bladder and kidney.
Can be fatal.
Body can cure all with this biomagnetic pair.

TEMPLE

At sides of eye

TEMPLE/TEMPLE
Special pair Isaac Cerebral microcirculation,
Pulmonary emphysema, Hypertension
Blood flow Temple/Temple can alleviate
bronchial tube problems.

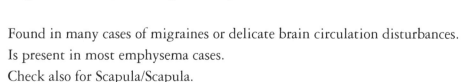

"Many babies die from muscular
tiredness of thorax (they can't breathe).
With preemies, use Temple/Temple and also
Scapula/Scapula and the ventilators are not necessary."
Regulation of cerebral and pulmonary flow.

Found in many cases of migraines or delicate brain circulation disturbances.
Is present in most emphysema cases.
Check also for Scapula/Scapula.

TEMPORAL
Above ear

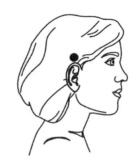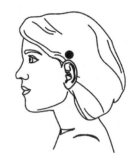

TEMPORAL/TEMPORAL
Typhus exanthematique virus
Main cause of migraines and
chronic headaches.
Transmitted by flea or rat bite.
Gives irritability,
nervousness, fever,
mental confusion,

LEFT TEMPORAL/LEFT TEMPORAL
Polyoma virus
From birds.
Respiratory infections
Potentially tumor causing

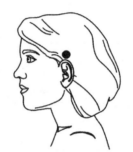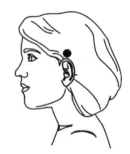

RIGHT TEMPORAL/CARDIA
Prion asylum / reservoir

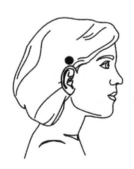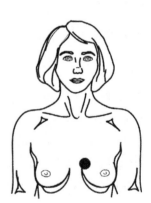

RIGHT TEMPORAL/RIGHT TEMPORAL
This is special pair "Bonilla" for
aggression
Many criminals found to have it.

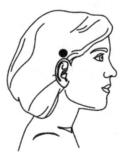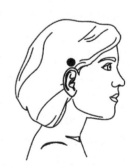

TENSOR

Tensor of the muscle going below greater
trochanter on
side of leg to foot on each side

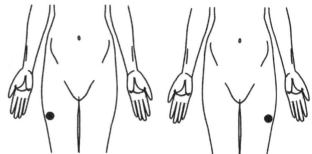

TENSOR/TENSOR

Giardinella vaginalis bacteria
Vaginal inflammation

TESTICLE

"Balls"

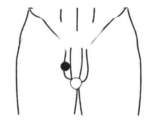
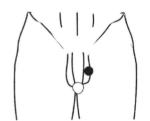

TESTICLE/TESTICLE

Yersinia pestis bacteria.
Is like Ovary/Ovary in women
If a woman has too much body or facial
hair, put magnets on her Testicle/
Testicle area.
Gives laryngeal bronchitis-type cough,
with vaginal flux in women and azoospermia in men
If Testicle/Testicle unbalanced in men, can give high voice.

THYMUS

Half way down and to right of sternum

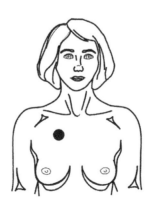
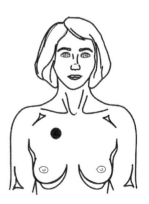

THYMUS/THYMUS

Glandular dysfunction
Sickness associated with thymus
Can come to be AIDS
Perhaps this gland is associated with
getting old.

THYMUS/ADRENAL
Special pair Alvaro Echeverria
Hormonal dysfunction
If you find this pair, check to see what
hormone is affected from:
Pituitary, pineal, thyroid,
parathyroid, adrenals, pancreas,
kidney, ovary, testicle.

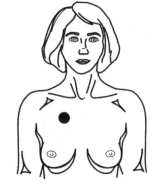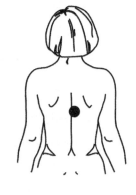

THYMUS/APPENDIX
Special pair Angeles
Improves white blood cell
production and quality and raises
lymphocytes

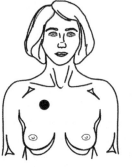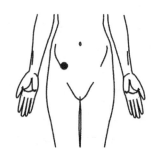

THYMUS/PARIETAL
Rubella virus
German measles
Headache, general malaise,
Eye hemorrhaging
Does not give immune deficiency.

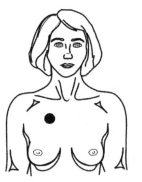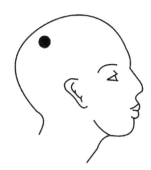

THYMUS/RECTUM
HIV 1 (AIDS)
Goiz says a bacterium gives AIDS
The virus is in the rectum,
and has a supportive role,
Affects production of thymus
hormones (CD3, CD4) as well as
T4 lymphocytes

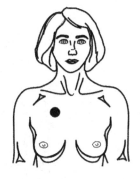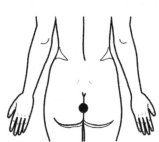

THYROID

At sides of Adam's apple

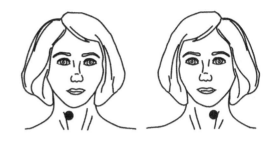

THYROID/THYROID

Glandular dysfunction
Check at sides or front of throat
Gives obesity, goiter,
exophthalmos, trembling hands,
liquid retention.

TIBIA

Inner, lower leg bone between knee and ankle
Magnets go close together, touching. Put
them between the two legs, one on each tibia.

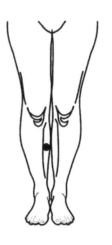
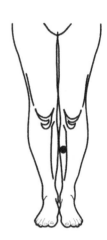

TIBIA/TIBIA

Pityrosporum (an obsolete name) fungus
or *versicolor or Malassezia furfu*r, very
aggressive fungus. This can end up
in gangrene and in losing a limb.
Can produce a cancer when
combined with another bacterium or virus.
Red coloration in skin,
Simulates scarlatina or
psoriasis (skin blotches),
ulcers in epithelium

TONGUE

The tongue is a large organ and
the points can be located all along
it. Check for placement from front of mouth
to back by angle. Put magnets on
outside, not inside of mouth.

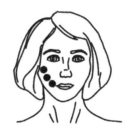
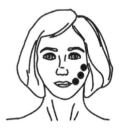

TONGUE/TONGUE

Scabies or mange parasite
Dermatitis-type skin problems.

Causes alopecia areata (hair falling out
by handfuls), is transmitted from animal hair.
Upon associating with another pathogen, can
give false tongue or larynx cancer

(Psoriasis can also cause alopecia areata).

TONSIL
Between commissures under chin

TONSIL/TONSIL
Herpes 2 virus
Associated with varicella (chicken pox).

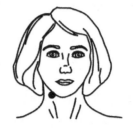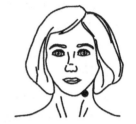

TRACHEA
Parallel to sternum on right or left
Put two magnets vertically
Both either on right or left of sternum

TRACHEA/TRACHEA
Influenza virus
Gives Rhinitis, sinusitis
Nasal disorders

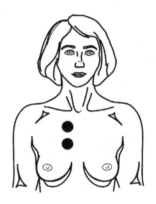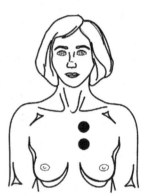

TROCHANTER, LESSER
Between legs, but angled

TROCHANTER, LESSER/ TROCHANTER, LESSER
HIV 3, HIV 4
Can be a reservoir of viruses

In a woman, is by the entry to vagina, as
high up on the legs as you can get, one on each side.
In male, is where prostate is so turn magnets to side
of legs also. Or can access this point at back of
legs under buttocks.

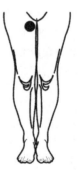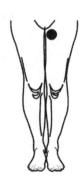

TROCHANTER, MAJOR

On outer part of hip bone—the part that
sticks out the most on the hip.

TROCHANTER, MAJOR/ TROCHANTER,MAJOR

Salmonella typhus bacteria
Common typhus, typhoid fever
Gives back pain,
digestive disorders diarrhea.
Main cause of false diabetes
mellitus, which is curable.

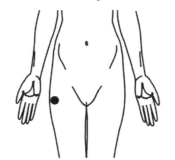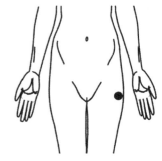

ULNA

Bone of forearm, little finger side

ULNA/ULNA

Herpes 3
Gives mucus in mouth or throat
Manifests internally
Associated with varicella (chicken pox)

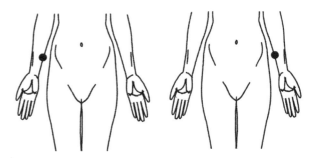

URETER

Above navel from navel to bladder
passes over peritoneum. Are on each side
of bellybutton

URETER/URETER

Varicella zoster virus causing chicken
pox, shingles and cystitis.
Constricts vessels and ureters
Polarizes positively one ureter and it
can go from navel to the bladder
(so as not to confuse it

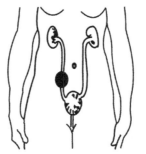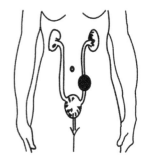

with ovary or Fallopian tubes) while the
other ureter is negative in charge.
In children, varicella is cutaneous.
In adults, it goes to ureter,
producing cystitis, bleeding and
ureteritis.

Is confused with urinary papiloma
In women, gives vaginal bleeding.
(Often these women get hysterectomies
and then they still bleed)
This also causes female infertility.

It can give lower back pain in adults,

The autonomic nervous system,
sympathetic and parasympathetic
run along the length of the spine
up to the neck and head area.
If a woman has a virus or bacterium
in this area (more common in women)
it can easily cause headaches, as the
pain runs up to the head.

URETHRA

Down by bladder above where legs join
Put magnets one above another

URETHRA/URETHRA
Corona virus
Transmitted by cats and rabbits
Is confused with renal insufficiency
Gives bloody discharge

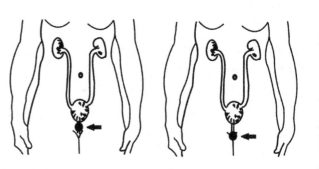

UTERUS
Above bladder

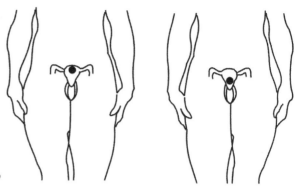

UTERUS/UTERUS
Special pair Roberta False pregnancy
Convenient to impact the pair
Can hide bacteria, or viruses such as
HIV, or a parasite If uterus is
positive-negative, could be a parasite.
This is a false pregnancy caused by a
parasite. This means that there may also
be endometriosis, so to rid uterus of micro organism, put the magnets on Uterus/Uterus,
with the negative one on top of the uterus, the positive one on bottom of uterus.

UTERUS/OVARY
Special pair Duran. Is powerful pair and care must be taken. Is pair for true pregnancy.

Situated in ovary donating fertilized egg and uterus.

If leg shortens with negative on uterus, take care. Goiz discovered that in a normal
pregnancy, a polarization or BMP is always formed between the uterus and the ovary
donating the ovule that becomes fertilized. It is a special magnetic bond that lasts for
and is intimately involved, maintaining the pregnancy for the nine months of gestation.
After delivery, the pair spontaneously disappears.
As soon as implantation occurs, the polarization shows up if a magnet is placed over the uterus.
The woman's leg shortens. If this occurs, Goiz recommends that the second magnet over the
ovary not be placed (as it would depolarize the pair) and tests be done to verify a true pregnancy.

VAGINA
Below bladder

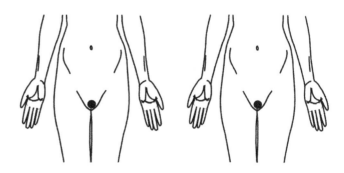

VAGINA/VAGINA
Yersinia pestis bacteria
Laryngeal bronchitis-type cough
With vaginal flux in woman and
Azoospermia in men

Can also be in Testicle/Testicle

VAGUS NERVE

On side of neck under
back of ear.

VAGUSNERVE/VAGUS NERVE

To lose weight
For digestion

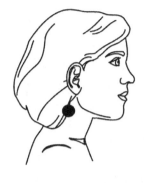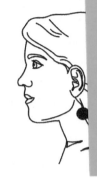

VAGUS NERVE/KIDNEY of opposite side

Special pair Benavides.
This is a universal reservoir of
viruses and bacteria.
Can negatively affect neurological
system.

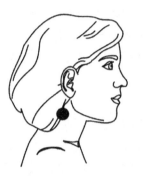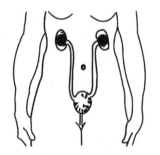

WRIST

Between hand and arm

WRIST/WRIST

Rickettsia bacteria
Indicates Alzheimer's if in combination
With Calcaneus/Calcaneus.
Gives symptomology from bellybutton
(waist) and up..
Children can have this.
It produces a toxin that goes to
the brain. (If not Alzheimer's, it can be
encephalitis, meningitis, Guillan
barre)

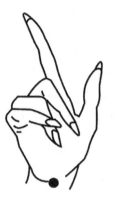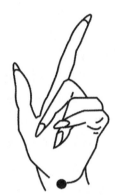

CHAPTER 19
APPENDIX

In line with Goiz's findings, another aspect of bioenergy came to light earlier in 1968 through the research, as mentioned, of Dr. Esther del Rio of Mexico. She noticed a powder-like substance on slides of animal tissue she was preparing. Most lab assistants making such slides, noting unknown contaminants, would simply wash them off, thinking they were careless in preparing the slides. However, Dr. del Rio knew she had taken scrupulous care creating her slides. Instead of washing off the contaminant, she, curious, checked the powdery nuisance under the microscope. What she found is being recognized for its importance in bioenergetics. For example, Cambridge University in England awarded her

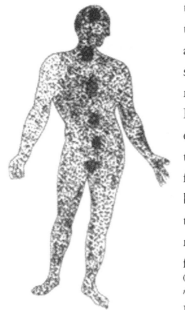

the title of "Woman of the Year" 1995-6. She discovered that the impurities were ferrous oxide and ferric oxide. "Minerals!" She realized they were from the tissue samples themselves and not from external foreign contaminants. These minerals form a magnetic substance known as magnetite. Ferrous and ferric oxide, or iron, is found in the body as part of hemoglobin (HEM), enzymes, flavoproteins, and ferroproteins. It is significant as it is united to many proteins in the form of macromolecules. In the case of HEM (in the red blood cells), the molecules are 3 dimensional in space in the form of pyramids. Dr. del Rio says our blood contains a myriad of magnetic pyramids. "The whole blood stream is full of resonances, vibrations, and electromagnetic energy." (Ariadna Gabriela Luce Gomez, "Energia Magnetica en el Cuerpo Humano," *Par Biomagnetico, Biomagnetismo Medico y Bioenergetica, Experiencias de Curacion, Ano 2005,* Vol II, p. 569)

In other words, hemoglobin not only carries oxygen from the air and carbon dioxide from the cells, it is involved in the electro magnetism of our bodies.

Our bodies contain numerous tiny particles of magnetite--around 100 million of them. They form a magnetic network from our head to our feet. Some areas of the body contain more magnetite than others, and Dr. del Rio, (in a private conference with this author) said that the areas of the chacras have the highest concentration of them. (See diagram)

Dr. del Rio cautions that in her research with the magnetite network composing our bodies, she has learned that if X rays or cobalt (radiation) are applied to the magnetite particles, they can be deactivated or totally destroyed. This disrupts our magnetic network, harming our health. She also stresses that since we are composed of levels of magnets, we need to care for this precious magnetite.

"Illness," she explains, "occurs when those magnets found in ferrous oxide and ferric oxide forms are disoriented. Often, the illness can be relieved simply by returning the magnetite to its place. This can be done without attacking the body with medicines, but simply by the applications of regulated magnetic fields." (See *Esther del Rio: Por las Venas Corre Luz*, p. 5)

Such application of magnetic fields ties directly in with what Goiz and his students carry out with magnets.

Information about acquiring magnets for use in Bioenergetic Basics techniques can be obtained from many sites on the internet. Due to certain restrictive laws in the United States, it is now not possible for the author to sell or promote the sale of magnets.

Keep in mind when ordering that the magnets should be natural magnets of at least 1,000 gauss and less than 50,000 gauss. Another option is to find a free source in your local area where microwave ovens and speakers are repaired. Very often the old magnets are discarded or given away at a low cost.
Best of luck!

PLEASE VISIT OUR WEBSITE WHERE WE POST NEW INFORMATION:

www.bioenergeticbasics.com

- Additional Information About Our Wellness Education Products
- Frequently Asked Questions
- Seminars, Events, and Appearances with Janice Bailey

For information on Janice Bailey's English translation of *El Par Biomagnetico*,

Contact: Basilio Perez # 11, Col. Constitution de la Republica
Mexico, D. F. C. P. 07469.
Internet: www.biomagnetismo.com.mx
E mail: biomag@mpsnet.com.mx

For information on the original Spanish version of *El Par Biomagnetico,*
Contact: Medicinas Alternativs y Rehabilitacion, S.A. De C. V.
Lucerna 62-7 piso.
Colonia Juarez C.P. 06600.
Mexico, D.F.
Internet: www.biomagnetismo.com.mx
E mail: biomag@mpsnet.com.mx

For additional research volumes (in Spanish) from the Center of Biomagnetic Medical Investigation,
Contact:

CENTRO DE INVESTIGACION DE BIOMAGNETISMO MEDICO,
S.C. at the Autonomous University of Chapingo in Mexico:
DIRECTOR GENERAL
Tel. 52 595 952 1500

PROFESSOR-INVESTIGADOR
Isaac Goiz Duran
Tel. 52 555 781 8511

Other Information in Spanish from the Colegio Mexicano de Biomagnetismo Medico, A.C.:   Tel. 52 555-591-1000

CHAPTER 20
BIBLIOGRAPHY

Bailey, Janice. "Experiencias y Exitos con el Par Biomagnetico." *Par Biomagnetico, Biomagnetismo Medico y Bioenergetica, Experiencias de Curacion, Ano 2006.* Vol. II. Isaac Goiz Duran and Guillerno Mendoza Castelan, editors. Mexico: Universidad Autonoma Chapingo; Programa Universitario de Medicina Tradicional y Terapeutica Naturista; Centro de Investigacion de Biomangetismo Medico, S. C., 2006.

_____. Personal collection of unpublished biomagnetic pair notes and information from private conversations, classes, seminars and conferences with Isaac Goiz Duran including those held: April, 2000; April 2002; April, 2003; January to November 2006; August, 2007, October, 2008; and October, 2009.

Balliett, Suzy. *The Complete Guide to Biomagnetic Therapy: Everything you need to know to create protocols, provide therapy and document outcomes.* Lyons, CO: Lazuli Press, 1996.

Becker, Robert O., M.D. *Cross Currents: The Promise of Electro Medicine, The Perils of Electropollution.* Los Angeles, CA: Jeremy P. Tarcher, Inc., 1990.

Becker, Robert O. and Gary Selden. *The Body Electric: Electromagnetism and the Foundation of Life.* New York: Quill, William Morrow, 1985.

Brown, William H. & Elizabeth P. Rogers. *General Organic and Biochemistry.* Boston: Willard Grant Press, 1980.

Childress, David Hatcher, ed. *Antigravity and the World Grid.* Box 74, Kempton, Illinois 60946, USA: Adventures Unlimited Press, 1995.

Cockrum, E. Lendell, Ph.D. *Rabies, Lyme Disease, Hanta Virus and Other Animal-Borne Human diseases in the United States and Canada.* Tucson, AZ: Fisher Books, 1997.

Coetzee, H., Ph.D. "Biomagnetism and Bio-Electromagnetism: The Foundation of Life," *Future History*, Series 1, Vol. 8. Los Gatos: Academy for Future Science, P.O. Box 35340, Menlo Park, 0102, Pretoria, South Africa, 1985.

Crossland, Alfreda. "New Hope Offered by Magnetic Therapies," *Journal of the Bio-Electro-Magnetics Institute,* Vol. 2. No. , Fall, 1990.

Eden, Donna with David Feinstein. *Energy Medicine.* New York: Jeremy P. Tarcher / Putnam, 1998.

Facklam, Howard and Margery Facklam. *Bacteria.* New York: Twenty-first Century Books, 1994.

Garcia Cuevas, Fernando Alberto. *La Globalizacion del Amor: Un Mensaje Acuatico.* Naucalpan, Mexico: Grupo Editorial Endira Mexico, S.A. de C.V., 2007.

Gerber, Richard. *Vibrational Medicine: New Choices for Healing Ourselves.* Santa Fe, New Mexico: Bear & Company, 1996.

Goiz Duran, Isaac, *Biomagnetic Pair, The.* Translated by Janice Bailey. Privately published. 2002.

_____. *Fenómeno Tumoral, El.* Loja, Ecuador: Editorial Universitaria de UNL, 2003.

_____. *Par biomagnetico, El.* Edo de Mexico C.P. 55310, Mexico: Medicinas Alternativas Y Rehabilitacion, S.A. de C.V., 1999.

_____. *Sida es Curable, El.* Mexico, D. F., Mexico: Intertipos Arias, S. A. de C. V., 1996.

Herrera, Catalina. *Esther del Rio: Por las Venas Corre Luz.* Mexico City, Mexico: Impresora Comercial S. A. de C.V., 1998.

Hills, Christopher. *Supersensonics: The Spiritual Physics of All Vibrations From Zero to Infinity.* Boulder Creek, California: University of the Trees Press, 1978.

Horowitz, Leonard G. *DNA: Pirates of the Sacred Spiral. Sandpoint, Idaho 83864: Tetrahedron Publishing Group, 2004.*

Jungreis, Susan A. "Biomagnetism: An Orientation Mechanism in Migrating Insects?" *The Florida Entomologist,* Vol. 70, # 2 (June 1987), published by the Florida Entomological Society.

Luce Gomez, Ariadna Gabriela. "Energia Magnetica en el Cuerpo Humano." *Par Biomagnetico, Biomagnetismo Medico y Bioenergetica, Experiencias de Curacion, Ano 2005.* Vol. II. Guillermo Mendoza Castelan and Isaac Goiz Duran, editors. Mexico: Universidad Autonoma Chapingo, Programa Universitaria de Medicina Tradicional y Terapeutica Naturista, Centro de Investigacion de Biomagnetismo Medico, S.C., 2005.

Molinare Pimentel, Tiare. "El Par Biomagnetico y el Hemisferio Sur," *Par Biomagnetico, Biomagnetismo Medico y Bioenergetica, Experiencias de Curacion, Ano 2006.* Vol. I. Guillermo Mendoza Castelan and Isaac Goiz Duran, editors. Mexico: Universidad Autonoma Chapingo, Programa Universitaria de Medicina Tradicional y Terapeutica Naturista, Centro de Investigacion de Biomagnetismo Medico, S.C., 2006.

Null, Gary. *Healing With Magnets.* New York: Carroll &Graf Publishers, Inc. A Division of Avalon Publishing Group, 1998.

Oldstone, Michael. *Viruses, Plagues, and History.* New York: Oxford University Press, 1998.

Philpott, William H. and Sharon Taplin. *Bio-Magnetic Handbook: A Guide to Medical Magnetics The Energy Medicine of Tomorrow.* Choctaw, OK: Enviro-Tech Products, 1990

Sitchin, Zecharia. *Cosmic Code, The.* New York City, New York: Avon Books, 1998.

Stoupel, Eliyahu, M.D., Ph.D. "Clinical Cosmobiology." *Newsletter of the Bio-Electro-Magnetics Institute.* Vol. 1: Number 1, Spring, 1989.

Tierra, Michael. *Biomagnetic and Herbal Therapy.* Twin Lakes, WI 53181: Lotus Press, 1997.

Van De Graaff, Kent and Stuart Ira Fox. *Concepts of Human Anatomy and Physiology.* Dubuque, Iowa: Wm. C. Brown Publishers, 1986.

Werner, David. *Donde No Hay Doctor: Una Guia para los Campesinos que Viven lejos de los Centros Medicos.* P.O. Box 1692, Palo Alto, CA 94302: La Fundacion Hesperian, 1980.

Young, Robert O., with Shelly Redford Young. *Sick and Tired? Reclaim Your Inner Terrain.* Pleasant Grove, UT: Woodland Publishing, 2001.

Zimmerman, John, Ph.D., and Dag Hinrichs. "Magnetotherapy: An Introduction." *Newsletter of the Bio-Electro-Magnetics Institute.* Vol. 4: Number 1, March 1995.

INDEX

Forehead 12, 118, 159, 163, 185
Frigidity 93, 137
Frontal 124, 159
Fungus 39, 40, 43, 45, 93, 158, 165, 174

Gait 93
Galactorrhea 185
Gall bladder 66, 93, 96-8, 102, 107, 117, 171, 201
Gall bladder duct 107
Gall bladder stones 93
Gangrene 93, 205
Gas See Flatulence.
Gastric insufficiency 93, 149
Gastric reflux 94, 179
Gastritis 75, 94, 101, 134, 162, 198
Gastroenteritis 94, 194
Gauss 1, 15, 16, 36, 56, 212
German measles (rubella) 91, 117, 126, 204
Giardia lamblia 89, 94, 111, 152
Giardinella vaginalis 78, 94, 124, 203
Gingivitis 94, 157, 174
Glandular disorders 94, 143
Glaucoma 94, 141
Gliosarcoma 94
Gluteus 103, 125, 135, 160
Goiter 94, 205
Goiz 1-4, 59, 60, etc.
Goiz special pair 59, 60, 181
Gonococcus 77, 152-53
Gonorrhea 53, 77, 79, 91, 94, 107, 112, 117, 122, 153, 157, 173-4
Groin 94, 132
Growth process 89, 94, 200
Guillan Barre virus 81, 88-91, 94, 111, 114, 116, 125, 185, 210

Haemophilus influenza 51-2, 88, 94, 96, 113, 139, 170
Hair, excess 94
Hair loss 94, 206
Halitosis 94, 179
Hand 14, 85, 89, 92, 104, 109, 113, 120, 143, 161, 210

Hands, trembling 95, 205
Hanta virus 95, 176
Headache 95, 111, 132, 137, 143, 148, 174, 197, 200, 202, 204, 208
Hearing 95, 155
Heart 60, 84, 95-6, 110, 112, 123, 134, 139, 148-50, 183, 195
Heart attack 95, 148
Heartbeat 60
Heartburn 95
Helicobacter pilori 50, 52-3, 78, 88-9, 94, 96-7, 100, 108, 119, 121, 123, 134, 162, 198
Hemorrhoids 96, 147
Hepatic abscess 96
Hepatic amoeba parasite 96, 103, 111, 172
Hepatic cirrhosis 96, 107, 116, 170
Hepatic duct 43, 80, 149
Hepatic faciola 83-4, 89, 155
Hepatic ligament 75-6
Hepatic, retro 122, 162
Hepatic syndrome 96
Hepatitis A 96-7, 101, 112, 125, 147
Hepatitis B 76, 83, 86-7, 91, 96, 101, 159, 187
Hepatitis C 96, 105, 172
Hepatitis D 96, 154
Hepatitis E 96, 102, 146-47
Hepatitis F 80, 96
Hepatitis G 97, 100-1, 104, 125, 147-48
Hepatitis H 80, 97
Hepatitis I 97, 189
Hepatitis J 97, 112, 189
Hepatitis K 97, 119
Hepatitis L 91, 97, 125, 172
Hernia, hiatus 97
Herpes 1 97, 125, 146
Herpes 2 52, 77, 97, 122, 206
Herpes 3 76-7. 82, 85, 87, 97, 101, 105, 108, 141, 207
Herpes 4 97, 140
Herpes 5 97, 103, 105, 148
Herpes 6 97, 104, 126, 166
Herpes 7 97
Herpes 8 97, 145

Made in the USA
Columbia, SC
18 July 2020

14096144R00141